Working with Staff to Overcome Challenging Behavior Among People Who Have Severe Disabilities

A Guide For Getting Support Plans Carried Out

Dennis H. Reid and Marsha B. Parsons

Volume 1
in
The Behavior Analysis Applications in Developmental Disabilities Series

Habilitative Management Consultants, Inc.

ISBN Number 0-9645562-3-5

Published by
Habilitative Management Consultants, Inc.
P.O. Box 2295
Morganton, North Carolina 28680

Professional Press
Chapel Hill, NC 27515-4371

Manufactured in the United States of America
04 05 06 10 9 8 7 6 5 4 3 2

DEDICATION

This manual is dedicated to the following people who have worked with the *Carolina Behavior Analysis and Support Center* over the years to help fulfill its mission of research, training, and consultation directed at increasing independence and life enjoyment among individuals with developmental disabilities: Carolyn Green, Leah Browning, Mary Hensley, Maureen Schepis, Perry Lattimore, Helen Reid, and Duke Schell.

ACKNOWLEDGMENTS

There are too many people who have influenced our writing to adequately acknowledge each individual contribution. However, several colleagues have been especially influential for one or both of us in regard to developing the content of this manual. In particular, we would like to acknowledge Jim Phillips, Gerry Faw, Martin Ivancic, and Phil Wilson for serving as models for how to work with staff to overcome challenging behavior among people with severe disabilities. We are fortunate to have had the opportunity to witness the clinical, supervisory, and consultative effectiveness of these professionals, as well as the pleasant and respectful manner in which they accomplished their duties with both support personnel and people with disabilities. Additionally, we would like to acknowledge David Rotholz for his help in teaching and refining our ideas and procedures through his collaboration in developing the *Carolina Curriculum on Positive Behavior Support.*

ABOUT THE AUTHORS

Denny Reid and Marsha Parsons have a combined total of more than 50 years experience in the human services. They have worked with support staff and people with severe disabilities and challenging behavior in a wide variety of residential, educational, habilitative, and vocational settings. Denny and Marsha have also provided consultative and training services in over 30 states, and collectively have published over 100 journal articles, book chapters, and books involving supervision and clinical applications in developmental disabilities. Two of their recent works, *Motivating Human Service Staff: Supervisory Strategies for Maximizing Work Effort and Work Enjoyment* and *Training To Teach In A Day*, are in their second printing and have been purchased by human service practitioners across all 50 states.

Denny is currently the Director of the Carolina Behavior Analysis and Support Center, and Project Director for the Leadership and Management Training Program of the Human Development Center of the Louisiana State University Health Sciences Center. Marsha is the Director of the Dogwood Resource Center of Western Carolina Center. Denny and Marsha reside with their respective families in Morganton, North Carolina.

TO CONTACT THE AUTHORS

Requests for consultative and training services from Denny Reid and Marsha Parsons should be directed to the address below. Readers are also invited to send comments about this manual, as well as ideas for future editions in the *Behavior Analysis Applications in Developmental Disabilities Series.*

Habilitative Management Consultants, Inc.
P. O. Box 2295
Morganton, North Carolina 28680

CONTENTS

SECTION I

INTRODUCTION TO WORKING WITH STAFF TO OVERCOME CHALLENGING BEHAVIOR AMONG PEOPLE WHO HAVE SEVERE DISABILITIES

SECTION II

CHARACTERISTICS OF A THERAPEUTIC ENVIRONMENT FOR PREVENTING AND TREATING CHALLENGING BEHAVIOR

SECTION III

SETTING THE OCCASION FOR EFFECTIVE IMPLEMENTATION OF BEHAVIOR SUPPORT PLANS: ESSENTIAL PROGRAM COMPONENTS AND STAFF TRAINING PROCEDURES

SECTION IV

MONITORING AND EVALUATING STAFF PROFICIENCY IN IMPLEMENTING BEHAVIOR SUPPORT PLANS

Chapter 9

SECTION V

INCREASING, MAINTAINING, AND IMPROVING STAFF PROFICIENCY IN CARRYING OUT BEHAVIOR SUPPORT PLANS

Chapter 10

Chapter 11

SECTION I

INTRODUCTION TO
WORKING WITH STAFF TO OVERCOME CHALLENGING BEHAVIOR AMONG PEOPLE WHO HAVE SEVERE DISABILITIES

CHAPTER 1

Working With Staff: A Critical But Overlooked Component in Overcoming Challenging Behavior Among People Who Have Severe Disabilities

One of the most difficult issues in the field of developmental disabilities is the prevention and treatment of challenging behavior. Although only a minority of individuals with developmental disabilities engage in challenging behavior of a serious nature, the behavior that is displayed by those individuals impacts many people. Challenging behavior affects not only the individuals who engage in the behavior, but also the lives of their peers, support personnel, and family members.

The harmful effects of challenging or problematic behavior are perhaps most evident with cases of self-injury and aggression among people with severe disabilities. Self-injurious and aggressive behavior results in serious bodily harm to literally thousands of people each year, and in the most extreme cases, death. However, there are also many other types of challenging behavior among people who have severe disabilities that if not treated effectively, have very harmful effects. The latter problem behavior includes for example, pica, property destruction, excessive water drinking, rumination, and extreme nonresponsiveness to social requests and expectations. Such behavior not only causes significant injury, it frequently results in individuals with severe disabilities being excluded from common societal functions and greatly detracts from an enjoyable quality of life.

In order to assist individuals with severe disabilities in overcoming challenging behavior, as well as to protect their peers and support personnel from the effects of the behavior, two general sets of procedures must be in place. First, there must be an effective treatment or support plan for preventing the challenging behavior from occurring, and for appropriately responding to the behavior if and when it does occur. Second, the treatment plan must be effectively implemented by all support persons who interact with the individual who engages in the problem behavior.

To effectively assist people with severe disabilities in overcoming challenging behavior, there must be a sound support plan *and* the plan must be implemented proficiently

In regard to the first issue just noted for overcoming challenging behavior, a tremendous amount of progress has occurred since the early 1970s in the development of effective treatment programs. In particular, the fields of applied behavior analysis and positive behavior support have developed a comprehensive technology for treating a very wide range of challenging behavior among people with severe disabilities. The technology has advanced to the point where a number of assessment procedures exist for determining what function different problem behaviors serve for a respective individual—that is, the individual's specific motivation for the behavior. Based on the results of various assessment procedures, the technology also includes numerous means through which support personnel can interact with an individual to alleviate the motivation for the problem behavior, and to assist the individual in attaining a desired outcome or function without a need for problem behavior.

The technological developments within applied behavior analysis and positive behavior support for preventing and treating challenging behavior represent one of the most influential advances in developmental disabilities in recent history. However, to date the actual impact of the developments on overall quality of life of people with severe disabilities and challenging behavior is far less than the potential impact. In most human service settings, the available knowledge and technology for preventing and treating challenging behavior is applied only in small part. In short, we know much more about overcoming problem behavior than what we routinely apply in the settings in which people with severe disabilities live, work, and play.

Numerous explanations can be offered regarding why support plans for challenging behavior are not carried out in accordance with the existing knowledge base and current technology. The primary reason though is that the advances resulting from applied behavior analysis and positive behavior support have occurred at a much faster rate than the ability of service personnel to determine how to incorporate the advances within the day-to-day routines of people with severe disabilities. In some cases, service settings such as group homes, day treatment centers, and sheltered workshops simply do not have the personnel resources to carry out currently recommended practices in regard to treatment plans for challenging behavior. At least equally frequently however, effective treatment is not provided because direct support personnel do not implement plans in the manner in which the plans are intended to be implemented.

The importance of the performance of direct support personnel in carrying out treatment plans for challenging behavior cannot be overestimated. In the vast majority of human service settings, direct support staff spend considerably more time with individuals with severe disabilities than any other agency personnel. Direct service personnel also are responsible for providing the major share of all supports and services needed by people with severe disabilities, and come into contact with challenging behavior far more frequently than anyone else in the service setting. Hence, in large part, if direct support personnel do not implement treatment plans in an appropriate manner, then there essentially is no treatment for challenging behavior for many people who have severe disabilities.

Difficulties in ensuring direct support personnel conduct treatment plans for individuals who have challenging behavior exist in human service settings throughout the United States. Problems with implementation of behavior support plans are reflected in a number of ways. In particular, lack of effective treatment resulting from insufficient program implementation has led to an over reliance on numerous types of medications to sedate or otherwise override the occurrence of challenging behavior. Such medications often have detrimental side effects for individuals with severe disabilities, and frequently do not address the actual reasons why people engage in challenging behavior. Poor program implementation has likewise resulted in individuals harming themselves or others, as well as an over reliance on restraint devices and procedures to protect individuals from harm—often in lieu of treatment. The occurrence of harm and overuse of bodily restraint has led to a number of agencies being cited by the United States Department of Justice for being in violation of the civil rights of the agencies' consumers.

If support personnel do not implement treatment plans proficiently, then in essence there is no treatment for challenging behavior

Probably the most pervasive indicator of the difficulties direct support staff experience in adequately implementing treatment plans for challenging behavior stems from reports by clinicians and related personnel who develop treatment plans. Interactions with clinicians in treatment and residential settings throughout the United States have indicated the biggest obstacle to effectively treating challenging behavior is nonproficient or inconsistent implementation of the designated plans. The professional literature is similarly replete with reports of difficulties in ensuring direct support personnel implement treatment plans appropriately.

The difficulties direct support staff experience in implementing designated treatment plans for challenging behavior should not be taken as a negative reflection of the people who work in direct support capacities. Rather, in the vast majority of cases in which problems with staff implementation of treatment plans exist, the reason for the problems is insufficient preparation of the staff and lack of day-to-day supervisory and clinical support for carrying out the plans. Direct service staff cannot be realistically expected to conduct treatment plans appropriately unless there is adequate preparation of the staff and subsequent support by management and clinical personnel. Implementing treatment plans for challenging behavior often is a time- and labor-intensive process, as well as a process that requires some rather complex interaction skills and careful timing of interactions. In order for direct service personnel to adequately fulfill these important duties in addition to their numerous other work responsibilities, they must be provided adequate preparation and support by management and clinicians on a routine basis.

It should not be expected that treatment plans for challenging behavior will be implemented proficiently unless there is strong management and clinical support for direct service staffs' implementation duties

Purpose of *Working With Staff to Overcome Challenging Behavior Among People Who Have Severe Disabilities*

The purpose of this manual is to describe how to work with human service staff to ensure proficient implementation of support plans for preventing and treating challenging behavior among people who have severe disabilities. In respective chapters, step-by-step procedures are described for ensuring that direct service and related personnel are equipped with the skills for implementing support plans, and then use those skills to carry out the plans consistently and effectively during routine work duties. The procedures to be described are intended to assist human service agencies in establishing and maintaining a work environment for staff that not only ensures treatment plans are carried out proficiently, but also reduces the likelihood that problem behavior will develop in the first place.

In considering the purpose of ***Working With Staff to Overcome Challenging Behavior***, it should be noted that the focus is on challenging behavior among individuals who have *severe* disabilities. The content is directed specifically for agencies serving people who have primarily profound, severe or moderate cognitive disabilities, autism, or highly significant multiple disabilities. These individuals present rather unique needs and issues for service providers relative to individuals with less pronounced disabilities (e.g., mild cognitive disabilities). In regard to the specific focus of this manual, the communication challenges and difficulties in acquiring adaptive skills that are characteristic of people with severe disabilities require special considerations for working with staff in a manner that effectively prevents and treats problem behavior.

Working with direct service staff to overcome challenging behavior among people with severe disabilities also requires special attention to the typical environments in which the latter individuals live, work, and play. Despite noted advances in including people with disabilities in normal community environments, most people with severe disabilities spend considerable amounts of time in congregate settings with other people who have special needs. People with severe disabilities constitute the primary population of public residential facilities for people with developmental disabilities (i.e., state institutions). Many people with severe disabilities also reside in congregate community settings such as group homes comprised of four or more individuals. Typical day treatment settings in which people with severe disabilities spend their weekday time are likewise of a congregate nature. To illustrate, despite advances in providing community-based, supported employment options for people with disabilities, the vast majority of individuals with severe disabilities who have obtained employment continue to work in congregate, sheltered workshops. For persons with severe disabilities who do not work, or work only part time, the most common day treatment settings are day activity programs and habilitation centers of a congregate nature.

Because most people with severe disabilities spend considerable amounts of time, if not most of their time, in congregate settings with other people with disabilities, the procedures for working with staff for overcoming challenging behavior discussed in this manual are aimed at congregate settings. These settings include residential agencies such as public and private institutions and group homes, as well as congregate day treatment settings including special education classrooms, sheltered workshops, and adult day activity centers. The focus is on preventing and treating challenging behavior in those settings in which there are *groups* of people with disabilities. Although many settings serving groups of people with severe disabilities are segregated from people who do not have disabilities, certain types of community inclusive environments also can involve groups of people with disabilities, albeit smaller groups relative to segregated settings. The latter settings, which are likewise addressed in this manual, include for example, various school classrooms and preschools. In these settings there may be two or more youth with severe disabilities along with typically developing children or adolescents.

Intended Audience of *Working With Staff to Overcome Challenging Behavior Among People Who Have Severe Disabilities*

This manual is intended for two primary audiences. First, the content is directed to supervisors and managers of direct support staff in congregate settings. This audience includes supervisors such as group home managers, residential unit and shift supervisors, lead teachers who supervise paraeducators, sheltered workshop supervisors, and supervisors in day activity programs. Second, the text is specifically aimed at personnel who are responsible for developing support plans for challenging behavior and to at least some degree, overseeing implementation of the plans. The latter individuals include psychologists, behavior specialists, behavior analysts, and team leaders such as Qualified Mental Retardation Professionals (QMRPs), Qualified Developmental Disabilities Professionals (QDDPs), and person-centered support team leaders. Administrative and executive personnel who have responsibilities for various components of the operation of residential and day treatment settings should also find the content useful and relevant.

Another audience for whom ***Working With Staff to Overcome Challenging Behavior*** is intended is advocates, family members, and program reviewers and evaluators. For this audience, the intent is to present procedural components that readers should expect to be in place in respective agencies if the agencies are to provide quality treatment programs for people with severe disabilities. The hope is that this audience will use information presented in subsequent chapters to assist agency personnel in designing environments that effectively prevent and treat challenging behavior. Relatedly, the hope is that an awareness of the information can be used to advocate for necessary changes where needed in order to help agencies improve their supports and services related to overcoming challenging behavior.

ORGANIZATION OF *WORKING WITH STAFF TO OVERCOME CHALLENGING BEHAVIOR AMONG PEOPLE WHO HAVE SEVERE DISABILITIES*

This manual is organized into six sections. In the remaining chapter in this section (**Chapter 2**), an overview of outcome management is provided. Outcome management represents a well developed means of working with personnel in human service agencies within a supervisory or consultative capacity. **Chapter 2** describes how the component procedures of outcome management represent a step-by-step means for working with staff to ensure support plans for challenging behavior are implemented proficiently and agency consumers achieve desired outcomes—in this case, overcoming challenging behavior.

In the second section of ***Working With Staff to Overcome Challenging Behavior***, procedures are described for establishing environments that help prevent challenging behavior from developing, and enhance treatment effectiveness if challenging behavior does occur. Respective chapters address the most important characteristics that constitute a therapeutic environment of a congregate nature for preventing challenging behavior. **Chapter 3** discusses the most fundamental characteristics of a therapeutic environment: individual safety. Common indicators of safe versus unsafe environments, and how these features affect problem behavior, are described in this chapter. In **Chapter 4**, the prevention of challenging behavior by promoting active engagement with the social and physical environment is discussed. Particular attention is directed to environmental characteristics that support people with severe disabilities in experiencing enjoyable lives. Life enjoyment is of course a major determinant of a desirable quality of life. Enjoyment with ones' daily life also reduces the likelihood of challenging behavior; people generally do not display problem behavior when they are enjoying themselves. Subsequently, **Chapter 5** describes how to prevent challenging behavior by teaching and supporting meaningful, functional skill development. Learning and using functional skills helps remove the need for people with severe disabilities to engage in problem behavior to fulfill their desires.

The third section of this manual presents procedures that specifically set the occasion for staffs' effective implementation of support plans for challenging behavior. The procedures described in this section represent what must happen before support plans are put in place in order to allow the plans to be effectively implemented by direct service staff. These procedures include ensuring the support plans have the essential clinical components to make the plans effective when implemented (**Chapter 6**), and means of training staff to implement the plans that guarantee staff will be skilled in carrying out all aspects of the plans during routine work activities (**Chapter 7**).

In the fourth manual section, procedures are described for efficiently yet carefully monitoring and evaluating staffs' implementation of support plans for challenging behavior. **Chapter 8** discusses the reasons why careful attention must be directed to monitoring of staffs' program implementation. **Chapter 8** also reviews general procedural considerations for ensuring monitoring is conducted not only effectively, but also in a way that supports a positive work environment for staff. A central theme in this as well as other chapters is that in order to establish a desirable environment for people with severe disabilities that effectively prevents and treats challenging behavior, the desirability of the environment from staffs' perspective must also be considered. **Chapter 9** then provides an in-depth summary of a specific means for monitoring the proficiency of staffs' implementation of support plans for problem behavior. The system described in **Chapter 9** can be used to observe and evaluate staffs' follow through with essentially type of support plan for challenging behavior.

The fifth section of this manual provides specific procedures for supporting and maintaining staff performance when staff are proficiently and effectively carrying out behavior support plans (**Chapter 10**), as well as procedures for improving staff performance when staff are not implementing support plans in an adequate manner (**Chapter 11**). The procedures for improving and maintaining staff performance as it relates to implementation of support plans for challenging behavior follow directly from information obtained from monitoring of staff performance as described in the preceding manual section.

Finally, in the sixth manual section, the **Appendix**, a form to be used to monitor and evaluate staffs' implementation of treatment plans for challenging behavior is provided. This section also includes **Selected Readings** that provide additional information for interested readers that relates to various topics addressed in preceding chapters. The **Selected Readings** likewise include references to much of the applied research upon which the content of this manual is based.

Preventing and Treating Challenging Behavior in Congregate Settings: An Agency-Wide Concern and Commitment

Before proceeding with the main content of ***Working With Staff to Overcome Challenging Behavior***, a critical tenet warrants highlighting: *the effective prevention and treatment of challenging behavior cannot be viewed in a singular manner as the responsibility of only one or some of an agency's personnel contingent.* Preventing and treating problem behavior has to be accepted as a shared responsibility of personnel throughout a respective human service agency.

The contention that essentially everyone in a human service agency has some responsibility for helping consumers overcome challenging behavior is based on a number of critical factors. First, as noted earlier, serious problem behavior has detrimental effects on many people, including individuals who engage in the behavior as well as their peers, support staff, and family members. Essentially anyone who interacts with a person who has problem behavior is likely to be negatively impacted by the behavior. As such, preventing and treating challenging behavior must be an agency-wide priority in service agencies of a congregate nature.

For any organization to adequately address a majority priority within its day-to-day operations—such as the prevention and treatment of challenging behavior—all staff within the organization must be aware of the priority and work collectively to address it. Organizations rarely meet their priority goals if the goals are only addressed on a partial basis by a select group of agency personnel.

The second reason that preventing and treating challenging behavior has to represent an agency-wide commitment is because of the variety and multiplicity of responsibilities that must be fulfilled if the treatment process is to be successful. As will be discussed in-depth in subsequent chapters, overcoming challenging behavior requires that environments be well designed and managed from a social, physical, and staffing perspective. Further, treatment plans must be developed with essential clinical components, and support staff must be well trained and supervised in carrying out the plans. To adequately fulfill all of these essential responsibilities, numerous personnel across various departments or sections within a given human service agency must have a concerned commitment. Administrative and financial officers must help arrange the fiscal resources to allow a therapeutic environment to exist for agency consumers. Human resource personnel must ensure that necessary staff are readily available and can be efficiently replaced or recruited as necessary. Skilled clinical staff must be available to develop sound treatment plans and supervisors must have the time and skills to support direct service staff in carrying out essential duties involved in treatment plan implementation.

A third reason for establishing agency-wide responsibility for helping consumers overcome challenging behavior is based on a pervasive problem in human service agencies of a congregate nature: treating problem behavior is usually assigned, or assumed to be, the responsibility of only one or a small group of people. There is a tendency, for example, to assume that problem behavior is the exclusive domain of the psychologist or a related clinician (behavior specialist, behavior analyst, psychiatrist, etc.). Among psychologists and related clinicians, there is likewise a tendency to assume that supervising staffs' implementation of behavior support plans is the responsibility of other personnel in an agency who are in designated supervisory roles over direct service staff. When responsibility is fragmented in this manner, there is little likelihood that all service components necessary for effective prevention and treatment of challenging behavior can be arranged and maintained.

In congregate settings for people with severe disabilities, the effective prevention and treatment of challenging behavior involves all components of an agency's operating structures and processes

Throughout this manual problems arising from a lack of agency-wide commitment and involvement regarding the prevention and treatment of problem behavior will be illustrated. Means of resolving the problems will also be described such that agencies can provide a comprehensive, well-coordinated, and effective means of helping people with severe disabilities overcome challenging behavior. Special considerations for respective types of personnel in congregate settings will be highlighted in regard to the most common issues related to their specific area of responsibility in an agency. For example, a number of chapters provide a separate section on special considerations for authors of behavior support plans. The primary point of concern here is that conscientious efforts must be made to involve all aspects of an agency's human resource pool in preventing and treating challenging behavior. Without such involvement, an agency will not fulfill its human service mission, and agency consumers will not receive the quality supports and services that their agency espouses to provide.

A Quick Start for Using This Manual to Evaluate and Improve Staffs' Implementation of Support Plans for Challenging Behavior

For those readers interested in obtaining information in order to quickly evaluate and improve staffs' implementation of existing treatment plans for challenging behavior, a *quick start* for using this manual can be obtained by skipping certain chapters and going directly to **Chapter 9**. The *quick start* process is especially designed for readers who have considerable experience in developing behavior support plans for challenging behavior, as well as for readers with experience in supervising the implementation of support plans.

As noted previously, the observation system described in **Chapter 9** (see also the copy of the observation form in the **Appendix**) can be used to evaluate staffs' implementation of essentially any support plan for challenging behavior. After careful application of the monitoring system, readers interested in a *quick start* can then go to **Chapter 10** for information on supporting and maintaining current implementation efforts that are occurring proficiently, and to **Chapter 11** for information on how to improve staffs' implementation performance if necessary. However, to gain a more complete understanding of working with staff to prevent and treat challenging behavior among people who have severe disabilities, it is recommended that readers then go back to other chapters as time permits.

CHAPTER 2

Outcome Management: A Step-By-Step Process for Supervising Implementation of Behavior Support Plans

It is well established that direct support personnel are charged with fulfilling a critical role in the human services. It is also well acknowledged, however, that people usually begin direct service jobs with little or no training in how to fulfill their important duties. The lack of training to function in a direct service capacity is a serious concern in regard to preventing and treating challenging behavior among individuals with severe disabilities. Most apparently, without adequate training in the skills necessary to implement behavior support plans, direct service staff are often ill equipped to help consumers overcome problem behavior. In a number of cases, staff also can inadvertently promote problem behavior among consumers if they are not well prepared in methods of preventing and responding to the behavior. Hence, effective ways of training staff in work duties related to implementation of behavior support plans must be available.

Staff training represents a vital step in the overall process of ensuring treatment plans for challenging behavior among people with severe disabilities are adequately implemented. As will be noted throughout this manual though, adequate staff training is only a beginning point for assisting direct service personnel in carrying out treatment plans for challenging behavior; the training must be followed by strong management support during the staffs' day-to-day interactions with consumers.

The importance of management support for ensuring proficient implementation of treatment plans was noted in **Chapter 1**. In short, without sound management support, it is highly unlikely that treatment plans will be implemented appropriately. When treatment plans are not implemented by direct service personnel in the way the plans are designed to be implemented, then generally there is no true treatment for challenging behavior.

This chapter summarizes a basic supervisory and consultative process for working with staff to ensure support plans for challenging behavior among people who have severe disabilities are carried out proficiently and effectively. The management process to be described, *outcome management*, has been developed through almost three decades of research and application in human service settings (see **General Summaries of Outcome Management** section in the **Selected Readings** for information related to the research and background development of outcome management). Relative to other approaches to working with staff in human service agencies, outcome management has by far the most established research base and application history to document its efficacy for supporting direct service personnel in adequately fulfilling their critical job responsibilities.

Before describing the component procedures of outcome management, special attention is warranted to the issue of who has responsibility for supervising staffs' implementation of treatment plans for challenging behavior. As discussed in the following section, for a variety of reasons confusion and disagreement often exist between agency supervisors and clinicians who develop treatment plans regarding the responsibility for ensuring the plans are carried out appropriately. Confusion and disagreement over supervisory responsibilities set the occasion for future problems in the way behavior support plans are implemented by staff. Hence, a primary issue that must be addressed before staff can be trained and supervised in implementing treatment plans for challenging behavior is *who* will be responsible for overseeing staffs' implementation duties.

Deciding Who is Responsible for Training and Supervising Staff Charged With Implementing Behavior Support Plans

Confusion or disagreement over responsibility for supervision of staffs' implementation of behavior support plans occurs in large part because of the manner in which congregate, human service settings operate. In almost every setting serving groups of people with disabilities, services are intended to be designed and coordinated through a team approach. Readers are undoubtedly experienced with, for example, interdisciplinary teams, person-centered planning teams, transdisciplinary teams, individual family service teams or Individual Education Planning (IEP) teams. Designing and coordinating services and supports using a team approach has come to be a hallmark of standard operating procedure in human service agencies.

Team-based services have many valuable attributes, and recommended practices currently espouse team involvement in the development and review of support plans for challenging behavior. However, team approaches to designing and delivering services also have some drawbacks. In regard to supervising staffs' implementation of behavior support plans, reliance on a team approach can cloud individual responsibility for overseeing implementation of the plans. As a result, it is often unclear precisely who is responsible on a day-to-day basis for training and supporting staff activities associated with implementation of treatment plans. Without a clear delineation of responsibility for supervising staffs' treatment duties, supervision is likely to be inconsistent, contradictory, or essentially nonexistent. In order to set the occasion for effective supervision, decisions must be made early in the development of support plans regarding who has the designated responsibility and authority for supervising staffs' implementation of the plans.

A first step in effectively supervising staffs' implementation of behavior support plans is determining *who* is responsible for the day-to-day supervision

From a pure management perspective, it is generally most effective if the person who has primary responsibility for developing a consumer's treatment plan also be the one who has the responsibility *and* designated authority for training and supervising staff assignments for implementing the plan. The advantages of this type of organizational structure for ensuring proficient staff implementation of behavior support plans will be illustrated in the following sections. For purposes here the point is that application of the component steps of outcome management for supporting staff implementation of treatment plans is more efficient and effective if one person develops the plans and oversees their implementation.

Although the situation in which one person has primary responsibility (along with authority) for developing support plans and then supervising implementation of the plans, the situation is actually quite rare in typical human service agencies. The more common process is that one person has essentially exclusive responsibility for developing support plans. These personnel typically include psychologists, behavior specialists, behavior analysts and QMRPs (who in this case develop individual consumer plans but do not have supervisory authority over direct support staff who implement the plans). Someone else has primary responsibility for supervising staffs' day-to-day implementation of the plans. The latter personnel typically include group home managers, residential team leaders or shift supervisors, treatment team leaders who supervise all team members including direct support staff, and workshop or center directors.

In the typical team structure as just summarized, responsibility and authority for supervising implementation of support plans for challenging behavior follow one of three models. First, a given person such as a psychologist develops a treatment plan, gives the plan to the staff supervisor and then the supervisor is responsible for overseeing staff implementation of the plan. This type of situation is common in community residential and day treatment settings in which the person developing the plan is not a full time employee within the specific setting (e.g., a consulting or contract psychologist).

In the second type of supervisory arrangement, a respective person develops the plan and then that individual shares responsibility with the staff supervisor for overseeing implementation of the plan. This situation is common in settings in which the person who develops the plan has a clinical role in an agency such as a behavior analyst, but is not in the designated supervisory chain of command over staff who have responsibility for implementing the plan. The latter supervisory arrangement is common in large agencies, such as a number of state-operated residential facilities.

In the third type of supervisory arrangement, a designated individual develops the plan but there is essentially no specification of who is responsible for supervising implementation of the plan. The latter situation can occur in any setting, but should not exist anywhere. Without specification of a supervisor for staffs' implementation of behavior support plans, a template almost certainly exists for serious problems with staffs' implementation of the plans. Again, the first step for ensuring staff adequately implement support plans for preventing and treating challenging behavior is to determine who is responsible for supervising staffs' implementation duties.

Once a decision is made regarding who is responsible for supervising staff performance related to carrying out treatment plans, then the component steps of outcome management can be used as the specific means of supervision. If one person has the designated responsibility such as a psychologist or staff supervisor (e.g., a group home manager or residential shift supervisor), then that person can implement each step of outcome management to ensure staff follow through with their treatment duties. If several people share supervisory responsibilities, then different steps of outcome management can be individually carried out by each person. Precisely how to divide the management responsibilities between the designated supervisors will be discussed in subsequent chapters. However, regardless of how the supervisory responsibilities are distributed, the specific expectations for supervising implementation of each behavior support plan must be made clear to each person involved in the supervisory process.

A Special Note on the Responsibility of Treatment Plan Authors Regarding Supervision of a Plan's Implementation

As just indicated, there are several ways that responsibility for supervision of staffs' implementation of behavior support plans can be arranged. The particular arrangement within each agency should be determined by the agency's organizational structure and the skills of respective supervisors and clinicians. Within any agency arrangement though, people who write treatment plans for challenging behavior should always assume at least shared responsibility for the manner in which the plans are implemented.

The rationale for authors of behavior support plans assuming some responsibility for overseeing implementation of the plans is several fold. Most apparently, the author of the support plan knows the most about the rationale for, and specific treatment procedures constituting, each component of the plan. As such, the plan's author is in the best situation to offer technical support to staff as they attempt to implement the plan. If the plan's author is included in the supervisory process, then supervisory and technical support can come from the same person. Such an arrangement represents an efficient use of agency resources, and can reduce contradictory direction provided to staff that often happens when two or more people provide the respective types of staff support. Relatedly, being actively involved in supervising staffs' day-to-day activities associated with implementing a support plan can afford the plan's author with excellent opportunities to closely evaluate the efficacy and practicality of the plan, and to make refinements where needed.

Authors of behavior support plans must assume some responsibility for, and actively take part in, supervising staff duties associated with carrying out the plans

---

Despite the advantages just noted, the process of authors of behavior support plans assuming responsibility for supervising staffs' implementation of the plans is frequently difficult. The difficulty exists for several reasons. First, people who typically write behavior support plans such as agency or consulting psychologists usually are not a regular part of the agency chain of command that involves direct support staff. Psychologists and related clinicians often have no supervisory authority over direct support personnel. Expecting psychologists to supervise staff duties associated with program plans for challenging behavior without having supervisory authority usually places the psychologists in a frustrating situation, and one that is likely to result in only intermittent success at best. Supervisory responsibility without supervisory authority usually amounts to no true supervision.

A second reason that involvement of treatment plan authors in the supervision of direct service staff can be difficult relates to issues of territoriality that frequently exist in human service agencies. Agency personnel such as group home managers, residential shift supervisors or charge nurses who are assigned the major responsibility for supervising the daily work performance of direct service staff sometimes resent the involvement of psychologists or other treatment plan authors in the supervisory process. In some cases, supervisors are concerned that sharing supervisory responsibilities makes the supervision process more complicated or inconsistent, which makes doing their jobs more difficult and less effective. In other cases, supervisors resent having to perform the bulk of supervisory duties (e.g., scheduling staff, resolving staff complaints, making daily duty schedules for staff) while the treatment plan authors have to carry out only limited supervisory duties yet still have the same level of authority as the regular supervisors.

The reasons just illustrated for the difficulties psychologists and other treatment plan authors face when assuming responsibility for supervising the performance of direct service staff may seem in one sense to be of little substance. Nevertheless, the reasons are quite real in many service settings. Numerous authors of treatment plans have experienced serious problems, for example, in working with staff to oversee their implementation of treatment plans due to lack of support or discontent on the part of the staffs' regular supervisor.

Problems with involvement of treatment plan authors in the supervisory process also exist in a number of situations due to the authors themselves. Personnel who are charged with developing treatment plans for challenging behavior usually must have advanced, specialized training in a professional discipline such as behavior analysis or positive behavior support. Treatment plan authors also must meet various licensing or certification requirements in most human service agencies. Rarely does the specialized training or licensing focus on preparing such clinical personnel in methods of supervising paraprofessional staff, or even raising expectations that such supervision should be their responsibility. Consequently, many authors of behavior support plans do not view supervision of staff work duties as their responsibility.

The contention here is that authors of treatment plans for challenging behavior *must* assume at least shared responsibility for the manner in which the plans are implemented. The rationale for this contention is based on the way in which services have to be provided for people with severe disabilities if the services are to be effective. To illustrate, in the field of psychology at large—which is the primary discipline through which most authors of treatment plans receive their training—the most common treatment approach involves a psychologist working directly with a client or patient in circumscribed, individualized therapy sessions. Psychologists generally see patients once a week or less for an approximate hour at a time. In contrast, for people with severe disabilities, treatment services are almost never effective if the services are restricted to an hour or so per week.

To effectively prevent and treat problem behavior among people with severe disabilities, treatment plans usually need to be in place throughout a person's waking hours. Further, the treatment procedures need to be effectively implemented by everyone who has frequent interactions with the individual, which is usually direct support staff. Again, this places a primary responsibility for carrying out treatment plans developed by psychologists with direct service staff.

When considering the manner in which effective supports and services are provided for people with severe disabilities, it becomes clear that authors of treatment plans actually have two consumer groups. Most obviously, the primary consumer is the individual with severe disabilities who engages in challenging behavior. Of essentially equal importance, the direct service staff who must implement the author's treatment plans also represent a consumer group of the author. The treatment plan author must directly affect what staff do during their routine work duties with individuals with severe disabilities in order to implement a treatment plan. If the author does not impact what staff do during their interactions with consumers who engage in challenging behavior, then the treatment plan cannot be implemented. Treatment plan authors must recognize from the outset that to help a person with severe disabilities overcome a problem behavior, the authors must help staff implement the plan. Working with direct service staff to carry out a treatment plan should not be viewed as an obstacle to effective treatment, but simply as part of the regular treatment process.

If authors of behavior support plans assume responsibility for supervising staffs' implementation of treatment plans—which many concerned authors do—then the most logical means of overcoming problems with lack of apparent supervisory authority would seem to be the arrangement noted earlier: the author would be designated by the agency as the supervisor of direct support staff. However, although such a solution is straightforward in concept, it is difficult to accomplish. Being the primary staff supervisor entails numerous responsibilities that have little to do with treatment duties due to the varied nature of a direct service job. In most cases, if psychologists or other treatment plan authors are assigned these responsibilities (e.g., recruiting, hiring and scheduling staff, training staff in various duties independent of treatment issues, covering staff absences), there would be little or no time for developing effective treatment plans. Additionally, many authors of behavior support plans have no interest or inclination to supervise the myriad of duties with which direct service staff are charged.

Working with staff to implement a behavior support plan for an individual with severe disabilities is as much a part of treatment as developing the plan itself

In short, in most cases treatment plan authors will be in a position of at best, shared supervisory responsibilities over the implementation duties of direct service staff. While this arrangement may not be the most effective from a pure management standpoint, it nevertheless represents the most common arrangement in human service agencies. It is incumbent upon authors of behavior support plans to find a way to work within that system in order to ensure that their treatment plans are implemented in the correct manner, and that consumers with severe disabilities receive the quality supports and services they are intended to receive. The following supervisory procedures encompassed within outcome management represent a means through which authors can effectively carry out their part of staff supervision.

Component Steps of Outcome Management for Supervising Staffs' Implementation of Behavior Support Plans

A primary advantage of outcome management relative to other supervisory procedures is that this particular approach involves a series of clearly defined, specific steps for supervisors and clinicians to take as a means of supervision. A noted problem with other popularized approaches to human service supervision or management is that the approaches fail to specify precisely what constitutes *supervision.* The latter approaches often include appealing slogans or cliches regarding management philosophies, but do not help a supervisor or clinician know what to do to ensure staff carry out their assigned duties in a quality manner.

In essence, effective supervision involves actively working to support staff performance that is observed to be of sufficient quality *and* actively working to change staff performance that is observed to be of insufficient quality. Outcome management provides a template regarding the specific actions supervisors and clinicians can take to accomplish these two essential aspects of effective supervision. This template, representing the component steps of outcome management, is provided in the following table.

COMPONENT STEPS OF OUTCOME MANAGEMENT

Step 1: Specify expected duties of staff

Step 2: Train staff in the performance skills constituting the expected duties

Step 3: Observe staff perform the duties during the regular work routine

Step 4: Provide positive support for staff performance observed to be adequate

Step 5: Implement corrective action for staff performance observed to be inadequate

---

Each of the component steps of outcome management just noted is summarized in the following chapter sections. Subsequently, individual chapters provide more detailed information regarding use of respective steps for effectively working with staff to ensure their implementation of support plans for challenging behavior is conducted proficiently and effectively. The purpose here is to provide an initial overview of outcome management.

Outcome Management Step 1: Specify Expected Duties of Staff

The first step in an outcome management approach to supervising staffs' implementation of a behavior support plan is to specify exactly what staff must do to carry out the plan. At first glance, this supervisory step appears rather straightforward; what staff should do to implement a consumer's support plan should be specified in the plan itself. Well designed treatment plans for challenging behavior make it very clear what must be done to prevent and treat a particular problem behavior. However, on closer examination it is apparent that many behavior support plans lack the degree of specificity that is necessary for staff to know precisely how they should interact and respond to a given consumer who displays problem behavior. Other treatment plans may contain the necessary specificity, but provide the information in a manner that is difficult or unrealistic for staff to obtain and comprehend.

In many cases, support plans for challenging behavior include sufficient specificity to allow staff to know how to carry out some components of the plans, but lack necessary information to carry out other aspects of the plans. A common example is a plan that specifies what staff should do when a respective consumer engages in problem behavior (e.g., interrupt the behavior and direct the consumer to another activity), but fails to specify what should be done to help prevent the behavior from occurring in the first place. For example, preventive measures included in support plans are frequently described along the lines of "keep the consumer busy". What it means for the consumer to be busy and exactly how staff can "keep the consumer busy" are not specified.

In cases such as the one just illustrated in which staff actions to implement a plan are not well articulated, it becomes highly unlikely that the plan will be carried out in the manner that the author of the plan intended. Different staff are likely to implement vague components of a plan differently. As will be illustrated in subsequent chapters, such a process not only compromises how the plan was intended to be implemented, but also can actually promote occurrence of the problem behavior.

There are numerous other examples of how support plans for challenging behavior lack sufficient specificity to allow well-intended staff to implement the plans appropriately. Information on how to evaluate a written support plan for necessary specification as well as how to make plans more specific when necessary is provided later (see in particular **Chapters 6** and **9**). The point here is that before staff can be effectively supervised in implementing a behavior support plan using outcome management, staff duties associated with the plan must be clearly specified. Such specification should come directly from the plan itself.

Although additional information for ensuring appropriate specificity exists in behavior support plans will be provided in the following chapters, there is a general guideline that can be helpful for all supervisors and authors of support plans to always keep in mind: *staff duties for implementing behavior support plans should be specified to the degree that supervisors and clinicians can observe staff performance and readily determine whether or not staff are implementing each step of the plan in the right manner.* Application of this guideline means that a supervisor or clinician can observe what staff are doing and immediately determine if their performance coincides with what should be done to prevent future occurrence of the behavior, or what should be done when a problem does occur.

A behavior support plan should be specified to the degree that supervisors and clinicians can enter staffs' work place and readily determine if each part of the plan is being implemented in the correct manner by direct service staff

Outcome Management Step 2: Train Staff How to Implement a Support Plan

If direct support staff are to be realistically expected to implement a support plan for challenging behavior in an effective manner, then the staff must of course know how to carry out the plan. Training staff how to carry out treatment plans represents the second step of outcome management for ensuring proficient implementation of the plans. The importance of training staff how to implement a support plan generally is well established among human service supervisors and clinicians who develop treatment plans. Some type of staff training usually occurs whenever a new treatment plan is developed for a respective consumer's problem behavior. However, the manner in which the training occurs is often inadequate to ensure staff truly know how to implement the plan during their day-to-day work duties.

If staff training is to be effective, the training process must achieve two outcomes. First, the training must make staff aware of the rationale for the treatment program and what the program is intended to accomplish. Second, the training must ensure staff acquire the skills to actually carry out each aspect of the plan in the correct manner. In an outcome management approach, the former outcome is achieved by providing staff with a certain knowledge base or relevant *verbal* skills. The latter outcome involves assisting staff in learning specific *performance* skills.

The way in which staff are frequently trained to implement support plans for challenging behavior usually is relatively effective for providing staff with relevant verbal skills regarding the rationale and intended purpose of the plan. Staff typically are brought together in a meeting format and a supervisor or psychologist reviews why the plan has been developed and what the plan entails. Following the meeting the staff generally have a good idea about the need for the plan and the overall purpose of the plan. However, this type of training or meeting format rarely provides staff with the necessary performance skills to adequately carry out the plan—the training does not ensure staff know how to do what is written in the plan.

In order to ensure staff truly know what to do to carry out a support plan for challenging behavior, staff must be provided with *performance-based* training. Performance-based staff training is a multi-step process that involves verbally describing what should be done to carry out a support plan, providing a written description of what should be done, demonstrating for staff precisely how to implement the plan and then letting staff practice implementing the plan with guidance from the staff trainer. A more in-depth description of how to conduct performance-based training to prepare staff to carry out behavior support plans is provided in **Chapter 7**.

In addition to performance-based training procedures, effective staff training must be *competency based.* Competency-based staff training means that the training is never considered to be complete until the staff trainer actually observes staff carry out the treatment plan in the correct manner; the staff must demonstrate competence or mastery in implementing the plan as part of the training process. A detailed discussion of competency-based staff training is also provided in **Chapter 7**. The point here is that unless a staff trainer observes staff carry out each component of a treatment plan proficiently, the trainer cannot be sure that the training has been effective.

Outcome Management Step 3: Observe Staff Implement a Support Plan

A critical part of effectively working with staff to ensure quality work performance in the human services is maintaining an awareness of how well staff are performing their routine work duties. The best way for supervisors and clinicians to maintain such awareness is to directly observe staffs' work performance on a frequent basis. Observing or monitoring staff work activities represents the third step in outcome management.

Routinely observing the work performance of staff is also a critical prerequisite for implementing the remaining steps of outcome management. Before steps can be taken to support staffs' proficient work performance in order to help staff continue to work in an adequate manner—in this case working to carry out treatment plans for challenging behavior—supervisors and clinicians must observe the performance to determine that the duties are being carried out proficiently. Relatedly, before steps can be taken to correct work performance that is not of sufficient quality, supervisors and clinicians must observe staffs' work activities to know that improvements are warranted (and to know precisely what staff need to improve). Observation of staffs' application of behavior support plans is also necessary to know if plans need to be altered in order to better assist consumers in overcoming challenging behavior.

Observing staff work performance in order to fulfill the purposes just noted requires specific skills on the part of supervisors and clinicians. The observations must be conducted in a fair and objective manner. The observations likewise must be conducted in a way that allows supervisors and clinicians to obtain an accurate and representative picture of the proficiency of staffs' routine activities associated with carrying out behavior support plans. Equally importantly, monitoring of staffs' work performance needs to be accomplished in a manner that staff find acceptable. Monitoring represents an event that staff often dislike, resulting in serious morale problems as well as inadequate work performance. Hence, monitoring of staffs' implementation of behavior support plans must be conducted in a manner that avoids discontent among staff.

Unless supervisors and clinicians are skilled in observing staff work performance in a manner that meets the just noted criteria, the observations will not allow for effective implementation of the other component steps of outcome management. Observations conducted without attention to the criteria also can cause much disgruntlement for staff as well as supervisors and clinicians. How to conduct observations of staff work duties in an effective and acceptable manner is discussed in-depth in **Chapter 8**. Subsequently, in **Chapter 9**, a monitoring procedure specifically designed for observing how well staff implement each component of a respective plan for a consumer's challenging behavior is presented. Use of the observation system described in **Chapter 9** can provide supervisors and authors of treatment plans with critical information regarding how to proceed with supporting or correcting staff performance for ensuring that treatment plans are implemented adequately.

Effective supervision of staffs' implementation of treatment plans for challenging behavior cannot occur unless supervisors and clinicians routinely observe staff carrying out the plans

Outcome Management Step 4: Support Proficient Implementation of Treatment Plans

Providing support for proficient implementation of treatment plans for challenging behavior is a critical but often overlooked component for ensuring plans are carried out in a quality manner. There is a natural tendency to believe that if things are going well—in this case, staff are doing a nice job of implementing treatment plans—no other supervisory actions are necessary. Such a belief and corresponding lack of action may suffice for a while, but inevitably leads to problems with program implementation in the long run.

Providing explicit support for staffs' proficient implementation of treatment plans must occur if the plans are to be consistently carried out in the appropriate manner. Direct service staff have many responsibilities to fulfill in human service agencies. Often, certain responsibilities compete with the time and energy necessary to carry out treatment plans for challenging behavior. Providing positive support for staff in regard to their program implementation duties can help ensure staff are aware of the importance of this aspect of their jobs, as well as help staff feel good about their successes in this area. Being well aware of the importance of a treatment responsibility and feeling good when work responsibilities are adequately fulfilled increases the likelihood that staff will continue proficient implementation of behavior support plans.

In addition to having many different responsibilities to fulfill, direct service staff frequently receive instructions and direction from many people. Staff are often given assignments, either formally or informally, by their immediate supervisor, agency executive personnel other than their immediate supervisor, and family members of consumers. Likewise, numerous clinical personnel expect direct service staff to carry out various clinically related duties. Nurses, teachers, and social workers, for example, frequently give instructions to staff concerning expected duties to complete. If personnel responsible for overseeing staff duties associated with implementing treatment plans do not provide sufficient support for the implementation duties, staff are likely to forego those duties in lieu of assignments given to them by other agency personnel.

Another reason supervisors and authors of treatment plans must provide support for staffs' appropriate implementation of program plans relates to the nature of providing quality treatment for challenging behavior. As indicated in the preceding chapter, preventing and treating challenging behavior among individuals with severe disabilities in congregate settings often requires considerable skill, patience, and effort. Unless staff are provided with sufficient support to facilitate these important duties, as well as to feel good about their accomplishments, staff are likely to lack the necessary motivation to continue exerting the effort needed to adequately carry out treatment plans.

In addition to the issues just noted, there is another more general reason why providing support for staffs' implementation of treatment plans is a critical step for ensuring the plans are carried out adequately. As will be discussed in the next section of this manual, an integral component in the prevention and treatment of challenging behavior among people with severe disabilities is ensuring that the environments in which these individuals live, work, and play is enriching and enjoyable. People, whether they have disabilities or not, are unlikely to display problem behavior if they have meaningful things to do and are enjoying themselves. In turn, it is not likely that the daily environments of consumers with disabilities will be enjoyable if the staff who work with the consumers in those environments do not experience an enjoyable quality of work life. By providing frequent supervisory support for staffs' duties associated with carrying out treatment plans, supervisors and clinicians can make at least one important aspect of staffs' work life more enjoyable.

If staff are to be expected realistically to provide an enriching and enjoyable environment for consumers with disabilities, then supervisors and clinicians must provide a meaningful and enjoyable work environment for staff

Effectively providing support for staffs' duties associated with carrying out treatment plans for challenging behavior involves two sets of supervisory actions. First, supervisors and clinicians must arrange the work setting and staff assignments such that implementing the plans is as easy as possible for staff. Second, supervisors and clinicians must frequently respond to staffs' implementation activities in a way that helps staff be aware of their successes and feel good about what they have accomplished. Specific steps supervisors can take to adequately provide staff support in each of these two ways is provided in **Chapter 10**. The procedures to be described in **Chapter 10** represent the most important supervisory and consultative responsibilities for ensuring that direct service staff work hard to carry out behavior support plans, carry out the plans proficiently, *and* enjoy their day-to-day work activities.

Outcome Management Step 5: Implement Corrective Action for Staff Performance Observed to Be Inadequate

By following the four steps of outcome management as just summarized, supervisors and clinicians will have a very effective means for helping direct service staff carry out behavior support plans in the way the plans are intended to be implemented. To briefly summarize, working with staff to ensure appropriate implementation of a behavior support plan begins by carefully specifying within the plan what staff should do to implement the plan. Next, staff should be trained in the skills to carry out the plan through performance- and competency-based training procedures. Staffs' day-to-day performance in implementing the plan should then be consistently and objectively observed in a manner that staff find acceptable. Following observations of staff carrying out their treatment duties proficiently, positive management support should be provided on a routine basis.

Application of these four outcome management steps consistently results in staff implementing behavior support plans proficiently and effectively. However, the success of this approach to working with staff should not be misinterpreted to mean that it is fool proof. The technology of supervising and consulting with human service personnel is by no means complete. At times, despite diligent and competent efforts by supervisors and clinicians, there will be occasions when respective staff do not carry out behavior support plans during their routine work duties in an appropriate manner. When observations (i.e., step three of outcome management) reveal problems with the performance of given staff related to implementation of behavior support plans, then supervisors and clinicians must take specific action to correct the problematic performance.

Taking corrective action to improve staff performance in implementing behavior support plans represents the fifth step of outcome management. This step is described in-depth in **Chapter 11** on corrective management. Corrective management involves specific ways for supervisors and clinicians to respond to observed inadequacies in staff performance related to carrying out treatment plans. In many cases, and especially if the first four steps of outcome management have been carefully followed, corrective action by supervisors and clinicians involves providing corrective feedback to staff regarding their performance. In a smaller number of cases, corrective management involves more significant supervisory responses such as disciplinary action. Again, these components of outcome management are described in **Chapter 11**. The point of concern here is that supervisors and clinicians must not let inadequate implementation of behavior support plans go uncorrected.

Section II

Characteristics of a Therapeutic Environment for Preventing and Treating Challenging Behavior

CHAPTER 3

Characteristics of a Therapeutic Environment for Preventing Challenging Behavior: Safety First

When initiating the support planning process for a person with challenging behavior, there is a tendency to focus on developing a treatment plan to intervene with the individual's behavior as quickly as possible. Once a serious problem behavior is observed, efforts tend to be directed to what can be done with the individual right away to stop or otherwise change the behavior. In the majority of cases though, this approach is not the most effective means of helping an individual overcome problem behavior. Instead of focusing initial treatment efforts on what can be done with the person, efforts should be directed whenever possible to what can be done with the *environment* in which the individual lives, works, or plays.

Challenging behavior among people with severe disabilities rarely exists without a reason, and that reason usually pertains to something associated with the surrounding environment. One's immediate social and physical environment can promote and support adaptive behavior as well as problematic behavior. Therapeutic environments set the occasion for the former behavior whereas nontherapeutic environments make it likely that problem behavior will occur.

Nontherapeutic environments influence the development and occurrence of challenging behavior in two general ways. First, an individual may engage in problem behavior as a means of *getting something* that the environment does not routinely provide. To illustrate, when congregate settings provide few opportunities for social interactions, consumers may seek attention from others through disruptive behavior. Second, an individual may develop problem behavior as a means of *getting out of something* that is occurring in the environment. A setting in which a consumer is frequently directed by staff to do something that the consumer does not like, for example, may lead to aggressive behavior as a means for the consumer to keep staff away and thereby avoid staffs' directives.

Because environments heavily influence the development and manifestation of challenging behavior, an initial focus of treatment planning should be to evaluate and, where necessary, improve the therapeutic quality of the environment. Attempting to treat challenging behavior in a nontherapeutic environment without addressing the problems within the environment almost always results in ineffective treatment; problem behavior cannot be treated in a problematic environment. In contrast, when an environment is truly therapeutic, not only is it less likely that challenging behavior will occur, it is more likely that treatment efforts will be successful if the behavior does occur.

Problem behavior cannot be treated in a problematic environment

Although there are different perspectives regarding what constitutes a therapeutic environment in congregate settings for people with severe disabilities, several characteristics generally are considered essential. In particular, environments must be *safe*. Individuals with severe disabilities must be assured reasonable protection from harm. Additionally, the environment must be *responsive* to consumers in terms of supporting or reinforcing interactions with the environment through participation in preferred activities. Environments must also be *habilitative* in nature by providing consumers with opportunities to learn useful skills—skills that enable them to live as independently and enjoyably as possible, and to fulfill their desires without engaging in problem behavior.

Preventing and treating challenging behavior is most successful in environments that are safe, responsive, and habilitative

In congregate settings, therapeutic environments seldom occur without planful, deliberate efforts to create and maintain them. Creating and maintaining environments that are safe, responsive, and habilitative is an ongoing process that usually requires frequent management attention. The supervisory and consultative procedures constituting an outcome management approach as summarized in **Chapter 2** are particularly suited to help supervisors and clinicians establish such an environment.

When using an outcome management approach to establish a therapeutic environment, the first step is to identify specific indicators that reflect whether the respective environment is therapeutic or not. Next, those indicators should be routinely monitored. If the indicators reveal that the environment is satisfactory, then efforts can be taken to support and maintain the environment. If the indicators reveal that the environment is not satisfactory, then corrective action must be taken to improve the environment.

The purpose of this as well as the following two chapters is to describe the primary characteristics of therapeutic environments. Within respective chapters, suggestions are offered regarding means for evaluating the essential characteristics of safe, responsive, and habilitative environments. Each chapter identifies variables common in congregate settings that detrimentally impact the therapeutic quality of an environment, and then suggests means for changing such variables. This chapter focuses on the most fundamental characteristic of a therapeutic environment, that of individual safety. **Chapter 4** discusses environmental responsiveness to support consumer involvement in preferred and enjoyable activities. **Chapter 5** discusses environments that promote consumer acquisition of meaningful skills that can replace the need for problem behavior.

Before discussing what constitutes therapeutic versus nontherapeutic environments, it should be noted that the conditions to be discussed rarely exist in total in any congregate, human service agency. Most agencies experience problems with one or more of the conditions at various times. Other agencies routinely experience difficulties with at least one of the conditions. Whenever one or more of the conditions to be discussed is problematic, the quality of consumer supports and services is likely to suffer and management action is warranted. Each condition also significantly impacts the effectiveness of support plans for challenging behavior.

The Most Fundamental Characteristic of a Therapeutic Environment: Personal Safety

The most fundamental concern in any setting providing supports and services for individuals with disabilities is personal safety. Individual safety represents a basic concern for all people, whether they have disabilities or not. Providing a safe environment is a special concern though in congregate settings for persons with severe disabilities.

Special concern for the safety of people with severe disabilities in congregate settings is warranted for a number of reasons. In particular, individuals who have severe disabilities are often unable to comprehend potentially dangerous situations, and are likely to have considerable difficulty communicating their concerns when they do recognize potential dangers. Additionally, many people with severe disabilities have difficulty protecting themselves from other persons who may engage in aggressive or other potentially harmful acts. These individuals also frequently have movement disorders or sensory deficits that increase their susceptibility to dangerous falls and accidents.

The importance of providing a safe environment for people with severe disabilities is well reflected in concerns expressed by family members. Personal safety is a primary criterion among family members in determining the adequacy of a congregate setting in which their relatives with severe disabilities receive supports and services. The importance of a safe environment is likewise apparent from a legal perspective, as numerous litigation cases and state as well as federal laws have asserted the legal right of people with disabilities to live in an environment that protects them from harm.

The importance of a safe environment also pertains directly to the prevention and treatment of challenging behavior. When individuals with severe disabilities are frequently hurt or afraid of being hurt, not only is their quality of life seriously compromised but the likelihood of problem behavior is increased. To illustrate, individuals are likely to respond with aggressive acts to protect themselves from other persons whom they fear. Being in a frequent state of worry or anxiety due to fear of harm also makes it more likely that an individual will respond to various environmental events with other types of problem behavior. Self-injury and disruptive behavior, for example, are likely to occur in order to change an environment that is perceived to be harmful. Such behavior has the effect of causing staff and other people present in the environment to change what they are doing in order to respond to the problem behavior. Many readers have likely experienced situations in which one consumer becomes upset or aggressive and then a "ripple effect" occurs through which other consumers become upset and engage in various types of problem behavior. The problem behavior among the latter consumers can function to protect them from the former consumer. Such behavior also can function to change the immediate environment by evoking certain responsive actions among support staff.

The most fundamental characteristic of a therapeutic environment is personal safety—people with severe disabilities must be guaranteed reasonable protection from harm and the fear of harm

In most congregate settings for people with severe disabilities, the essence of a safe environment is that consumers are protected from harm through provision of support commensurate with each consumer's needs, and consumer health concerns receive appropriate attention. Though these conditions may seem rudimentary, human service agencies continue to exist around the United States that do not uniformly guarantee even these most basic elements. Numerous reports of serious harm and injury among individuals residing in state institutions occurred across the United States throughout the 1980s and 90s. Once more individuals with severe disabilities began moving to community living sites of a congregate nature, increased incidents of physical harm and injury began to be reported in those settings as well.

Indicators of a Safe Environment

If human service agencies are to guarantee a safe environment for consumers with severe disabilities, the agencies must have objective measures for determining environmental safety. To obtain these measures, agencies must first determine meaningful indicators of safety, as well as a lack thereof, in a particular environment. Once indicators of safe and unsafe environments are identified, management systems can be designed and implemented to support the former environments and change or improve the latter environments.

In agencies serving groups of individuals with severe disabilities, a common indicator of environmental safety is the frequency of consumer accidents, and especially accidents resulting in physical injury. Although all congregate environments for people with severe disabilities ideally would be accident free, accidents and injuries are a part of life. Hence, agencies should have a systematic means of documenting and studying these events when they do occur.

Although accidents inevitably are going to occur in any congregate setting, accidents resulting in serious injury can be all but eliminated with careful planning and attention. The accident documentation process within an agency should include objective criteria for separating minor injuries from more serious ones. For example, an accident resulting in a slight scratch on the arm should be differentiated from one resulting in a broken bone. The number and level of severity of injuries should be summarized and reviewed by management at regular intervals. Comparisons of accident and injury data over time within the same agency, or to other agencies serving consumers with similar needs, provide one important indicator of environmental safety.

Certain events that do not result in apparent physical injury, but have a likely potential for resulting in harm, should also be reflected in an agency's monitoring system for accidents and injuries. These events, which are often referred to as some type of *unusual incident*, can reflect the safety of an environment because of the likely occurrence of an injury in the future if the events persist. An individual becoming lost or being left unsupervised for a longer than reasonable period of time represent examples of potentially harmful incidents that usually need to be documented. Documentation and subsequent scrutiny of events that potentially could result in serious harm can help managers recognize and alter problematic situations before injuries occur.

In addition to accidents and injuries, and situations that could potentially lead to injuries, indicators of environmental safety can relate to more general health concerns. The indicators of consumer health which are most important in a given agency are dictated by the characteristics and needs of the agency's consumers. To illustrate, many people who are nonambulatory require intermittent repositioning to relieve pressure on the skin. For these individuals, the frequency of inflammation or actual skin breakdown can be a critical indicator of environmental safety. In settings where a number of individuals receive medication, an important safety indicator can be the frequency of medication errors (e.g., wrong medication given to an individual, medication administered at the wrong time). Other examples of indicators relating to general health concerns include the frequency or duration of infectious illnesses, falls within various locations (e.g., bathroom or front steps of a group home), environmental cleanliness, health-related equipment failures, and consumer ingestion of nonedible substances.

The frequency of events resulting or potentially resulting in injury as well as general measures of health and well being represent indicators of environmental safety

Establishing a Safe Environment

If indicators of environmental safety reflect an unsatisfactory level or trend, management must carefully examine variables that may be contributing to the unsafe conditions. There are any number of variables that can impact the safety of an environment depending, in large part, on the aspect of safety in question. However, in typical congregate settings for people with severe disabilities, unsafe environments are frequently the result of one or more specific problem areas. The most common of these problem areas are presented below.

COMMON PROBLEM AREAS RESULTING IN UNSAFE CONDITIONS IN CONGREGATE SETTINGS INVOLVING PEOPLE WITH SEVERE DISABILITIES

- **Inadequate staff-to-consumer ratios**
- **High consumer density (crowding)**
- **Lack of staff familiarity with consumers**
- **Inappropriate staff deployment**
- **Absence of onsite staff supervisor**
- **Frequent staff absenteeism or turnover**

Inadequate Staff-to-Consumer Ratios

An adequate number of staff must of course be present in a respective setting to ensure that consumers receive appropriate health care and are protected from harm at all times. In residential settings, for example, there must be sufficient staff to ensure that the health and safety of consumers can be guaranteed not only from 8 a.m. to 5 p.m., which represents the time period when most human service staff are present, but also during the evenings as well as on weekends and holidays. Evenings, weekends, and holidays are of particular concern because staff-to-consumer ratios are usually lower at those times than on regular weekdays. When an unexpected staff absence occurs during these time periods, staff-to-consumer ratios can quickly fall to dangerously low levels.

Guidelines for desired staff-to-consumer ratios have been established by several licensing agencies for residential and educational settings that provide supports for people with severe disabilities. However, the most appropriate ratio of staff-to-consumers ultimately must be determined by the individual needs of the consumers in a given environment. A number of consumer characteristics should be considered in determining necessary staff-to-consumer ratios. When consumers are heavily dependent on staff for assistance with personal care for instance, higher staff-to-consumer ratios are needed to ensure environmental safety. More staff are likewise required in settings where several staff are needed to lift individuals for bathing, toileting, or repositioning than in settings where consumers can accomplish these tasks independently. Settings supporting consumers with serious problem behavior who require nearly continuous supervision to prevent them from harming themselves or others need more staff than settings where consumers have few problem behaviors. The more intensive supervision necessitated by consumer dependence or problem behavior must be provided in addition to, and not at the expense of, adequate supervision of other consumers in the setting.

An important step for avoiding serious problems that may arise from inadequate staffing patterns is to review staff work schedules *prior to* when staff are expected to be at work. It should also be noted though that the ratio of staff-to-consumers depicted on a written work schedule does not always provide sufficient information for judging the potential for an unsafe environment. When reviewing the number of staff scheduled to work as a means of determining staff-to-consumer ratios, it may not be readily apparent that the number of staff available to supervise consumers will likely fluctuate due to individual consumer needs and activities. Mealtimes, transportation, personal care routines, or problem behavior can affect the actual number of staff available to ensure the safety of all consumers present in a given environment. If one staff person is needed to take a consumer to a doctor's appointment or to work, for example, the actual number of staff available for supervising the remaining consumers can be seriously reduced relative to what is reflected on the staff schedule.

Instead of relying exclusively on the number of staff as indicated by a work schedule to determine the adequacy of staff-to-consumer ratios, frequent observations in the environment should be conducted to observe the number of staff available to directly supervise consumers at any given time. The *actual* ratios—that is, the number of staff and consumers observed in the setting at respective points in time—are usually a more useful means of determining whether or not staff-to-consumer ratios need improvement.

When judging the adequacy of staff-to-consumer ratios in a given environment, direct observations in the environment are needed to accurately determine the actual number of staff available to provide appropriate levels of support

High Density

A second variable that frequently impacts safety in congregate situations is the density of individuals in a respective setting. Density refers to the number of people present within a given physical space, or the amount of crowding. Although staff-to-consumer ratios may appear adequate based on numbers of people, if too many individuals are living or working in too small a space, the ability to protect consumers from harm can be compromised. In short, the more crowded a given space is, the more likely it is that harmful events will occur.

Some licensing agencies provide formulas for determining the maximum level of density for a given space. For example, the Title XIX Medicaid regulations for Intermediate Care Facilities have historically restricted the number of consumers with mental retardation who share a bedroom (typically a maximum of four individuals per bedroom). Even when the overall density in a respective environment conforms with a specified standard though, density can be a problem at certain times of the day or in specific parts of a building. To illustrate, density may be a problem in the living room of a group home at times when consumers tend to congregate for certain activities, or when consumers are waiting near a door in preparation to leave for work each morning.

In most cases, specific criteria for identifying likely problems with density are not readily available. Consequently, determining if density is creating a safety risk often requires repeated observations to count the number of people in specific locations in association with reported accidents and potentially harmful incidents. If a high number of accidents or safety-compromising incidents repeatedly occur at specific times or locations, density should probably be reviewed in those situations. Steps may then have to be taken to reduce the number of consumers in the respective locations at certain times.

The more crowded a given space becomes, the more likely it is that consumer safety will be compromised

Lack of Staff Familiarity With Consumers

The familiarity of staff with individual consumers has a major impact on personal safety in any congregate setting. People with severe disabilities depend on staff to help accomplish many activities of daily living. Because consumers with severe disabilities are likely to experience difficulty in communicating their needs, staff must be sufficiently familiar with consumers to know critical information about appropriate medical care, behavior support plans, preferred and nonpreferred items and events, requirements for supervision, and daily routines.

When a staff person is unfamiliar with consumers due to being new to the job, for example, unsafe situations can result. Most importantly, unfamiliar staff often have difficulty communicating with individuals who have severe disabilities and do not readily express themselves in conventional ways. Consumers can become upset, frustrated, or angry when unfamiliar staff do not understand or appropriately respond to the consumers' communication attempts. Consumers also can become upset when their daily routine is disrupted because a new staff person is unfamiliar with the daily schedule, or a serious accident may occur when consumers are not supervised as closely as necessary by a new staff person.

When environmental safety indicators reveal problematic situations, the degree to which staff are familiar with consumers usually warrants review. Subsequent sections of this chapter provide additional information regarding common situations that warrant management attention because the situations result in staff being unfamiliar with consumers and potential safety risks.

When staff are not familiar with individual consumer needs, unsafe situations ultimately arise for consumers

Inappropriate Staff Deployment

Another variable influencing environmental safety is the manner in which support staff are deployed. Satisfactory numbers of staff and consumers in a given environment will not guarantee the environment is safe unless staff are providing adequate consumer support. Ensuring staff provide the necessary support usually requires that staff be held accountable for completing certain work duties in specific locations. To adequately fulfill work responsibilities across various locations while maintaining safety for all consumers, how staff are deployed to complete their work duties warrants management attention.

Deploying staff to provide appropriate consumer support can be difficult because of the variety of duties that direct service staff are expected to fulfill. In addition to generally supporting and supervising consumer activity, these staff routinely have record-keeping and housekeeping duties as well programmatic responsibilities associated with individual consumers. With such varied responsibilities, it is not always clear to staff which responsibilities are the priority at any given time. Staff may inappropriately prioritize housekeeping or record-keeping duties over direct support duties involving face-to-face interactions with consumers. Management may likewise place pressure on staff to complete record-keeping duties to avoid problems with licensing and certification requirements. Excessive focus on such duties often reduces staffs' ability to oversee the safety of consumers relative to duties that involve interactions and close involvement with ongoing consumer activity.

The lower priority given to responsibilities involving direct contact with consumers relative to other types of tasks that do not involve interactions with consumers often occurs because the latter duties (e.g., making a bed, writing a note in a consumer's record) result in an immediate outcome that is readily apparent to staff, supervisors, and agency evaluators. In contrast, the positive outcomes of direct support responsibilities such as teaching a skill to a consumer or encouraging consumers to participate in a leisure activity are not always immediately apparent. It is incumbent on supervisors and clinicians to communicate the importance of support duties involving direct interactions with consumers, stressing that consumer supervision is always a priority.

To help organize staff time to complete various work duties including consumer support and supervision responsibilities, it is often useful to prepare detailed work schedules for staff. Structuring staff work time through scheduling serves a number of beneficial functions. As discussed in **Chapter 2**, clearly specifying staff work duties (which is a part of establishing work schedules) sets the occasion for staff to perform their jobs in a satisfactory manner. Detailed work schedules communicate to staff where they should be and what they should be doing during their work shift. Additionally, when work duties are clearly specified for individual staff members, then *supervisors* will know exactly what staff should be doing at any given time and in what location. Such knowledge among supervisors facilitates effective monitoring of staff work performance, which is another critical step of effective supervision and management (see **Chapters 8** and **9**). When it is clear to both staff and supervisors where staff should be and what staff should be doing at respective times during the day, staff can readily be held accountable for completing assigned duties and ensuring consumer safety.

Detailed work schedules clarify expectations for staff, assist supervisors in monitoring staff performance, and generally help hold staff accountable for fulfilling their work responsibilities

Absence of Onsite Staff Supervision

A frequently overlooked variable in providing a safe environment is the physical presence of a staff supervisor. The presence of a supervisor can affect environmental safety in a number of ways. Supervisors who are highly familiar with the day-by-day routine in a setting can make informed decisions as to whether an adequate number of staff are on hand, how those staff should be deployed, and whether staff are fulfilling their job duties to provide optimal support for consumers. Relatedly, when supervisors are present in an environment, they can respond immediately to the need to rearrange staff assignments, planned activities, or consumer groupings as may be required to alter a potentially unsafe situation. Supervisors who are onsite expedite such decisions because staff clearly understand who is "in charge". When supervisors are not present, it is often unclear who is responsible for making timely decisions, with a common outcome of no one taking charge to remedy a potentially problematic situation.

With the high amount of staff turnover encountered in many congregate settings serving people with severe disabilities (see next chapter section), there are likely to be inexperienced staff in direct support roles at various times as well as staff who are unfamiliar with a given group of consumers. An important safeguard is lost when a supervisor is not present to oversee the decision-making of less experienced or familiar staff that may impact the safety and well being of consumers. Moreover, inexperienced and unfamiliar staff may not be as aware as they should be about specific conditions likely to affect the safety and welfare of consumers. Onsite supervisory presence is likewise important because some staff—inexperienced or otherwise—tend not to work as diligently when there is no supervisor present. When staff begin to perform their support duties in an incomplete or otherwise inadequate manner, maintaining consumer safety becomes a risky venture.

Although there are numerous benefits of having supervisors present in staff work areas, having a supervisor present onsite at all times can be difficult if not impossible in many congregate settings. In settings providing residential services, for example, the number of supervisors working in an agency often is at a minimal level during evenings, weekends, and holidays. Additionally, supervisors who are on duty may be responsible for many settings (e.g., different group homes or residential units) and can be present in any one setting only briefly if at all. Agencies that provide supports and services for a small number of individuals in different settings with only one or two staff on duty at a time likewise encounter problems with onsite supervisory presence. In the latter agencies, having a supervisor routinely present is not very practical from a financial perspective because agencies simply cannot afford to employ that many supervisors.

Because an onsite supervisor can affect many aspects of staff functioning and consumer safety, an agency should consider alternative forms of supervision when maintaining an onsite supervisor is not practical. In particular, when a supervisor has responsibility for several sites, the supervisor should arrange to be at each of those sites several times each day. Frequent, unpredictable observations, or "spot checks", within each setting represent a reasonable alternative to continuous, onsite supervision. If supervisors cannot visit a site on a daily basis, then professional or clinical staff who may be intermittently present in the setting could be asked to conduct observations and report the results to the supervisor (see **Chapter 8** for detailed information on means of conducting monitoring checks in an appropriate manner).

A key predictor of whether supports and services are provided in the manner in which they are intended to be provided is the frequency with which a supervisor is present in staffs' work site; the more frequently a supervisor is present, the more likely it is that supports and services will be provided in the desired manner

Staff Absenteeism and Turnover

Two problems pervasive in many congregate settings where support personnel are employed 24 hours a day, seven days a week, are high rates of staff absenteeism and turnover. All of the variables contributing to an unsafe environment mentioned thus far are exacerbated to some degree by staff absenteeism and turnover.

Absenteeism and turnover almost always result in decreases in staff-to-consumer ratios. Relatedly, when staff absences occur, problems with density can arise because of the common practice of combining groups of consumers into one group so that a decreased number of staff can provide supervision (e.g., if a staff member assigned to a group of consumers on one side of a group home is absent, that staff person's consumer group may be sent to the other side of the house where staff are present, thereby doubling the density on the latter side of the house). Excessive turnover and absenteeism also often result in newly hired staff being assigned responsibility for consumer supervision before they have gained sufficient familiarity with consumers. Additionally, when staff are absent, supervisors may be required to perform the missing staff person's work, which leaves less time for fulfilling critical supervisory duties.

One common method for responding to staff absenteeism and turnover that often causes more problems than it resolves is temporarily reassigning or *pulling* staff from one part of an agency to another location in order to cover the job duties of an absent staff member. While pulling staff may appear to be a reasonable solution to providing staff coverage, the process usually creates both short- and long-term problems. In the short-term, reassigned staff must struggle to fulfill the needs of individuals with whom they have little familiarity. The area of the agency from which staff have been pulled also must operate without the optimal number of staff present. In the long-term, because staff frequently report that they intensely dislike being pulled from their routine work setting to cover the workload of others, the practice may actually increase turnover and absenteeism due to staff dissatisfaction with agency practices.

Because of the problems that result when staff are pulled from their routine work station to cover the work duties of an absent staff member, the practice of pulling should be used judiciously. Agencies plagued with high rates of staff turnover and absenteeism should seek long-term solutions to these problems. Guidelines for tackling these complex management issues are beyond the scope of this text; resolution of turnover and absenteeism problems usually requires comprehensive, agency-wide initiatives of a sustained nature. The interested reader is referred to the **Selected Readings** for additional information on staff absenteeism and turnover in the human services (see section on **General Summaries of Outcome Management**). The point of concern here is that when safety indicators in a given environment reveal problems, the frequency of absenteeism and turnover, as well as "pulling" staff to or from a setting, may warrant investigation.

In summary, safety should be the cornerstone of any environment in which individuals with severe disabilities live, work, and play. To ensure consumer safety, agencies must develop means for ongoing measurement of indicators of environmental safety and lack thereof. When environmental safety appears to be problematic, common situations affecting environmental safety as described in this chapter should be carefully reviewed and where necessary, rectified.

KEY PREDICTORS OF A SAFE ENVIRONMENT

1. **Adequate staff-to-consumer ratios exist consistently across all operational hours as reflected through direct observations in respective settings**
2. **Situations in which large numbers of consumers are gathered into a restricted amount of space are avoided**
3. **Staff providing consumer supervision are thoroughly familiar with individual consumer needs**
4. **Detailed work schedules that delineate consumer support duties are prepared by supervisors and followed by staff**
5. **A staff supervisor is frequently present in the environment**
6. **Staff absenteeism and turnover are maintained at low levels**

Special Considerations for Authors of Behavior Support Plans

Although the environmental conditions described so far in this chapter have been discussed in regard to personal safety of individuals with severe disabilities, the conditions also relate to the effectiveness of support plans developed for challenging behavior within congregate settings. The conditions should be considered by clinicians who develop treatment plans from two vantage points. First, several of the conditions warrant particular attention when attempting to determine the variables that occasion the occurrence of problem behavior. Second, certain conditions deserve consideration because they affect the likelihood that support plans will be implemented in an appropriate manner. How the conditions affect the prevention and treatment of challenging behavior will be covered in large part in subsequent chapters. However, there are several key issues related to specific environmental considerations that warrant highlighting here.

Staff Ratios

The primary issue concerning staff ratios for authors of behavior support plans is whether there are sufficient numbers of staff to realistically carry out a plan that is developed. If a support plan is designed in a manner that goes beyond the capability of staff to implement the plan because of insufficient numbers of staff, the plan will not be carried out consistently or effectively. Psychologists and other authors of behavior support plans must consider the typical staff resources in a given setting when designing a plan to make sure that the plan can indeed be carried out.

Designing support plans for challenging behavior in light of the available staff to implement the plans is a critical practical consideration. A common complaint among supervisors and direct service staff in a number of congregate settings is that support plans are designed in a manner that is impossible to carry out given the usual number of staff on duty and their other responsibilities. Developing treatment plans in consideration of available staff resources can also present a serious dilemma for authors of plans. The dilemma is that at times, authors have good ideas regarding how to treat a respective problem behavior but also know that what is needed for effective treatment goes beyond the capacity of the available staff in a given setting. Authors must decide whether to design the most effective plan that they can—which in this case is not likely to be carried out proficiently due to lack of sufficient staff—or to design a plan with less procedural features that is more likely to be amenable to staff implementation but likely to be less effective.

The dilemma just noted is faced by essentially every clinician who develops support plans at one time or another. Unfortunately, often there is no quick solution to the dilemma (see **Chapter 6** for additional discussion on this and related dilemmas for authors of behavior support plans). At a minimum though, authors of treatment plans should be aware of the typical staff resources, and be prepared to express this type of dilemma to agency management and negotiate where possible for increased (or re-assignment of) staff resources. This type of dilemma represents another reason why responsibility for treatment of challenging behavior has to be shared across different personnel within a given human service agency, including agency management in charge of staff resource allocation as noted earlier.

When considering the issue of availability of staff for implementing behavior support plans, it should also be noted that it can be difficult to determine if the issue is real or not. For a variety of reasons, in certain settings various staff do not carry out treatment plans under the guise of lack of time or resources. In these cases there really is a sufficient number of staff but staff simply do not want to exert the time and effort necessary to carry out support plans. When authors of support plans, in conjunction with appropriate supervisory personnel, determine that the issue is not one of insufficient staff resources but poor staff motivation, then adequate implementation of the plans becomes a serious management issue. Subsequent manual sections address how to overcome lack of motivation to secure necessary staff compliance in carrying out their treatment duties (see in particular **Chapters 10** and **11**).

Density

The primary issue with density for authors of support plans pertains to assessing the variables that affect the manifestation of challenging behavior. When consumers spend time in crowded places, problem behavior is likely to occur. High density or crowding can lead to problem behavior for numerous reasons. Some consumers become upset and display aggressive, disruptive, or self-injurious behavior simply because they are uncomfortable with peers being too close to them. In these cases problem behavior can function to help them escape the crowded situation by, for example, a support person escorting them to another, less crowded location when problem behavior occurs. Other consumers become upset because they receive less attention in crowded spaces due to other consumers seeking and receiving a greater portion of staff attention.

In many situations, density is an issue only during certain times of the day or in specific locations as illustrated earlier in this chapter. Thorough assessments (see **Chapter 6**) by authors of support plans can usually identify these particular situations, with subsequent ideas for helping staff and consumers avoid them. In other cases, such as in certain residential units or classrooms, there is almost a constant state of high density—there are simply too many individuals assigned to respective units or classrooms. In the latter situations, much more comprehensive changes are needed to alter the existing environment. Such situations should be identified by treatment plan authors before attempting to put a specific treatment plan in place because unless the environmental crowding is reduced, the plan is not likely to be effective.

Unless features of nontherapeutic environments are improved, there is little reason to develop a behavior support plan for an individual consumer; the plan is not likely to be effective in a problematic environment

Staff Familiarity With Consumers

Staff familiarity with individual consumers is a critical consideration in the development and implementation of behavior support plans. If staff are not familiar with a respective consumer due, for example, to having been pulled from another location within an agency, they are not likely to be sufficiently knowledgeable about the consumer's support plan. If staff are not aware of what constitutes a treatment plan, there is little likelihood of them carrying out the plan appropriately.

In many settings, and particularly residential settings, lack of staff familiarity with certain consumers almost always occurs from time to time. In other settings, staff unfamiliarity occurs essentially daily. In the former settings, authors of support plans usually must assume the responsibility of ensuring that the occasional unfamiliar staff is provided with sufficient training regarding a consumer's support plan as quickly as possible. In the latter settings, more comprehensive, systems change types of procedures are necessary. It is generally the responsibility of agency management to make the necessary systems changes to reduce problems with lack of staff familiarity with consumer needs. However, it is also the responsibility of treatment plan authors to make sure appropriate management representatives are aware of the issue, and also aware that there is little chance of a treatment plan being effective unless the problem is resolved.

Staff Deployment

Where and how direct service staff spend their work time has a direct impact on how well treatment plans are implemented. If staff are not in locations where plans need to be implemented or do not carry out each component of a plan in the appropriate manner, treatment is obviously going to be compromised. Both of these issues are primarily a supervisory responsibility, involving both the staffs' regular supervisor and the author of the treatment plan as referred to in the preceding chapter. Later chapters in this manual focus in greater detail on how to ensure staff are adequately deployed and sufficiently supervised to facilitate proficient implementation of behavior support plans.

Onsite Presence of a Supervisor

Earlier it was mentioned that a frequently overlooked variable affecting the safety of a congregate setting for people with severe disabilities is the presence of a supervisor in staffs' work environment. Supervisory presence is likewise a frequently overlooked factor affecting the proficiency with which staff carry out behavior support plans. Essentially all of the problems encountered in maintaining environmental safety in the absence of a supervisor also exist regarding staffs' proficient implementation of behavior support plans.

In short, staff are more likely to carry out their treatment-related duties appropriately if their supervisor is present on a frequent basis. In regard to authors of treatment plans, staff are also more likely to implement a plan proficiently if the author is frequently present. **Chapter 2** stressed the importance of treatment plan authors assuming some responsibility for staffs' implementation of the plans that they write. If such supervision is to be effective, the authors must be frequently present in staffs' routine work area.

The importance of authors of behavior support plans being frequently present in staffs' work area cannot be over emphasized. Being available onsite to offer technical assistance, oversee program implementation, provide encouragement for staff, and to generally trouble shoot is usually the one means for enhancing implementation effectiveness over which a clinician has almost total control. Psychologists and other treatment plan authors who take the time and effort to visit staffs' work area numerous times during the week also tend to be much more respected and accepted by support staff than authors who are rarely present. When staff respect and accept a clinician, the clinician's ability to impact staffs' implementation of treatment plans is enhanced considerably.

A critical variable affecting how staff implement a behavior support plan is how often the author of the plan is present and available in staffs' routine work area; the more frequently the author is present the more likely it is that the plan will be carried out in the correct manner

Staff Absenteeism and Turnover

Just as with establishing a safe environment, staff absenteeism and turnover are important to people who develop behavior support plans because these factors affect every environmental condition related to treatment plan effectiveness. This is an area though in which authors of treatment plans usually have little direct control. Nevertheless, when these events occur often, authors must make sure appropriate management representatives are well informed regarding how the factors may be compromising the prevention and treatment of challenging behavior.

A Final Note On Environmental Safety: The Environment Must Be Safe for *Everyone*

The focus of this chapter has been the safety of individuals with severe disabilities in congregate settings. However, environmental safety pertains to *everyone* in the settings. Peers or friends without disabilities who may be in the settings as well as agency staff must be safe. Safety, and the feeling of being safe, is particularly important for direct support personnel.

There are many features of congregate settings for people with severe disabilities that impact the safety of direct support staff. For example, environments in which many consumers are nonambulatory and require frequent lifting and transferring by staff pose a risk for back injuries to staff due to repeated or improper lifting. More relevant for the purpose of this text though, environments in which there is a high potential for aggressive behavior among consumers often present a risk of harm to direct support staff.

Staff concerns about their safety due to aggressive behavior among consumers result in numerous detriments for staff and consumers. Most apparently for staff, their quality of work life is seriously hampered when they are frequently worried about being hurt. As noted throughout this text, staffs' quality of work life has a direct impact on the quality of life of the consumers with whom staff work. For consumers, staff who are worried about being hurt experience difficulty fulfilling their support duties with consumers in a quality manner. Staff may tend to stay away from consumers whom they fear. Staff may likewise carry out their support duties in a hurried or incomplete manner in an attempt to minimize contact with certain consumers to reduce the risk of injury.

Ensuring staff work in a safe environment and are not anxious or worried about being hurt depends on the specific factors in a setting that affect the staffs' safety. In some cases, concerns over safety are due to a lack of sufficient staff to allow fulfillment of support duties and implementation of behavior support plans in a safe and proficient manner. In other cases, concerns over safety occur because adequate treatment plans do not exist to help consumers overcome problem behavior, or staff are not adequately trained to implement the plans.

It is the responsibility of agency management to ensure that staffs' work environment is safe and that staff feel safe while at work. It is likewise the responsibility of authors of behavior support plans to spend sufficient time with staff to determine if staff feel safe in regard to working with consumers who display dangerous or potentially dangerous behavior. Support plan authors should be vigilant about detecting safety concerns among staff, and work with appropriate management representatives to alert them to the concerns and help determine what can be done to resolve safety issues.

CHAPTER 4

Promoting Meaningful Consumer Activity Within Group Situations

Chapter 3 discussed the most fundamental characteristic of a therapeutic environment for people with severe disabilities in congregate settings, that of personal safety. This chapter focuses on the second most fundamental characteristic: consumer involvement in activities. Frequent participation of consumers in meaningful and enjoyable activities is a hallmark of quality service settings for people with severe disabilities.

The degree to which consumers participate in activities affects the therapeutic nature of a congregate setting in a number of ways. In particular, when a person actively interacts with the social and physical environment, the individual has opportunities to learn and develop new skills. Frequent participation in activities likewise provides opportunities for individuals to use and expand skills that have been previously learned.

Consumer activity also affects the therapeutic quality of a congregate environment from an individual enjoyment perspective. Actively interacting with the social and physical environment increases the likelihood that individuals will enjoy themselves on a day-to-day basis. In contrast, if an environment is void of activities in which consumers can participate, then typically consumers experience little enjoyment with their daily routine. The latter environments are characterized by frequent consumer boredom and general lethargy.

Congregate settings that fail to promote consumer activity not only interfere with individual learning and enjoyment, but also contribute directly to the development of problem behavior. People naturally need and seek stimulation from their surrounding environment. If a respective setting does not provide stimulation through opportunities to interact with the social and physical environment, then problem behavior often develops as a means of obtaining stimulation. It is well established, for example, that when an individual with severe disabilities spends much time in a barren or otherwise unstimulating environment, the individual may learn to obtain stimulation through stereotypic or self-injurious behavior. A person may similarly learn that engaging in aggressive or disruptive behavior can make an environment more stimulating. In the latter case, the problem behavior increases stimulation by causing support staff to interact with the individual in order to interrupt the behavior.

In addition to affecting the development of problem behavior, an environment that fails to promote consumer activity involvement impacts the *treatment* of problem behavior that does develop. To illustrate, a frequent component of many behavior support plans for challenging behavior among people with severe disabilities is to interrupt the behavior when it occurs and redirect the individual to an activity. If no activity is ongoing when the problem behavior occurs, there is nothing to which the consumer can be redirected. If staff create an activity in which to involve the consumer after the problem behavior has occurred, staff could easily reinforce or strengthen the very behavior they are attempting to treat by providing a potentially desired event whenever the behavior occurs.

Supporting people with severe disabilities to participate in activities enhances consumer learning and enjoyment as well as the prevention and treatment of challenging behavior

Because of the importance of individual activity involvement, the degree to which consumers with severe disabilities participate in activities has long been considered a primary means of evaluating the therapeutic quality of a congregate setting. However, consumer involvement in activities in and of itself does not ensure that environments will optimally support learning, enjoyment, and the prevention or treatment of problem behavior; the *types* of activities in which consumers participate also must be considered.

Many congregate settings for people with severe disabilities attempt to promote consumer activity involvement. The type of activity that is often encouraged though adds little to the therapeutic quality of the environment because the activity tends to have little meaning or enjoyment for the consumers. For a variety of reasons that will be noted later, individuals with severe disabilities in congregate settings are frequently prompted or expected to engage in the same activities day in and day out. The latter activities can quickly become repetitive and of little value to consumers. In other cases, the activities designed for consumers are based on what leisure items or games support staff have immediately available, with little or no bearing on what activities the consumers prefer.

When consumers are frequently presented with activities that have little meaning or enjoyment, the activities can cause more problems than they prevent. Most notably, repeatedly encouraging consumers to engage in meaningless or nonpreferred activities can increase the likelihood that challenging behavior will develop. Problem behavior occurs because it helps consumers to get out of something they do not want to do (e.g., throwing materials or striking staff when presented with activities that are disliked). From the perspective of direct support staff, repeatedly trying to involve consumers in activities that appear to have little meaning can be disheartening for the staff, and subsequently detract from staffs' willingness to attempt to promote consumer activity involvement.

Congregate settings that are truly therapeutic for people with severe disabilities support frequent consumer involvement in *meaningful* and *enjoyable* activities

In short, the involvement of consumers in activities that are meaningful and enjoyable is a critical feature of a therapeutic environment. It should also be noted though that maintaining a high level of consumer activity is often a very difficult undertaking in congregate settings for people who have severe disabilities. Many individuals with severe disabilities lack sufficient communication skills to request activities or to initiate appropriate interactions with others. Instead, they must wait for support staff to provide activities. Additionally, once provided things to do, some consumers lack skills to sustain engagement in the activities. As a result, the individuals frequently are highly dependent on support staff to arrange and maintain appropriate interaction with the surrounding environment.

Adding to the difficulty of promoting meaningful and enjoyable activity among people with severe disabilities is the typical ratio of staff to consumers in congregate settings. In most congregate settings, there are more consumers than staff. When consumers outnumber support staff, ensuring that all consumers are consistently involved in desired or meaningful activities requires considerable effort and diligence by staff.

Despite the difficulties usually inherent in supporting consumer involvement in meaningful and enjoyable activities, such support must occur if congregate settings are to provide therapeutic environments that enhance the prevention and treatment of challenging behavior. The purpose of this chapter is to describe how to effectively structure and maintain an environment to promote consumer involvement in meaningful activities. Initially, methods for identifying indices of beneficial consumer activity will be discussed. Specific procedures for monitoring and evaluating the indices subsequently will be described. Finally, some basic issues warranting consideration in order to enhance activity involvement where necessary will be presented.

Identifying Important Indicators of Consumer Activity Involvement

From an outcome management perspective, the first step in ensuring that an environment promotes consumer participation in meaningful activities is to identify valid indices of activity involvement. The intent is to specify what constitutes desirable consumer activity to the point that agency supervisors and authors of behavior support plans can enter a congregate setting and quickly determine the extent to which consumers are involved in the activities. To adequately make such a determination, the indices of consumer activity should allow for easy differentiation of the meaningful quality of different types of activities that are likely to be observed.

Differentiating the Quality of Activities

People can interact with the environment in many different ways. As noted earlier, some activities through which individuals with severe disabilities interact with the environment are more therapeutic than other activities. Generally, the types of activities in which consumers participate in congregate situations can be viewed as a hierarchy, ranging from activities that are the most therapeutic to activities that have essentially no therapeutic utility. The following figure illustrates such a hierarchy.

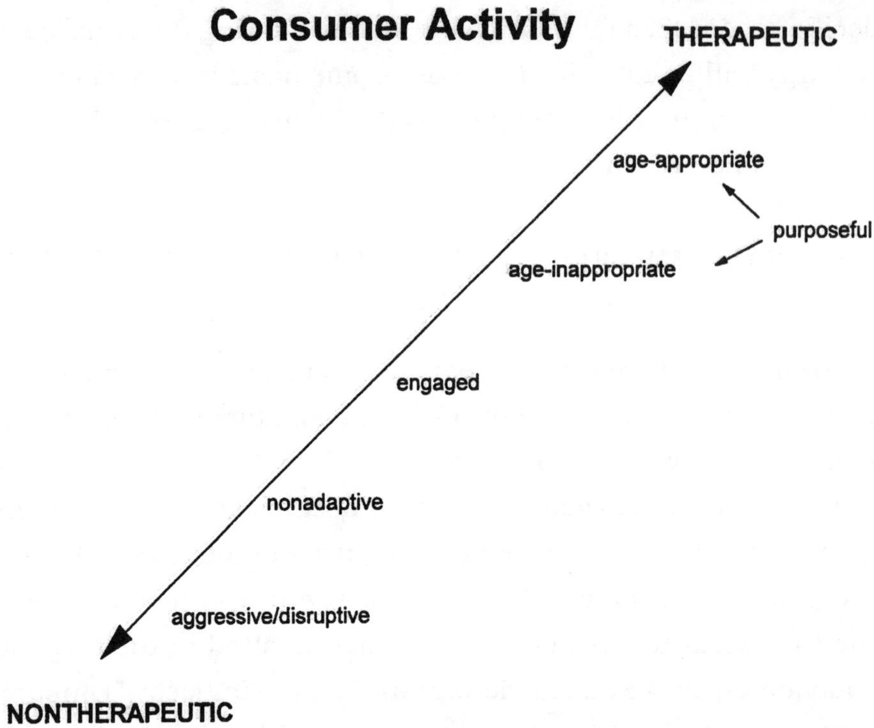

Figure 4-1: Hierarchy of therapeutic nature of activities in which people with severe disabilities participate in congregate settings.

Before describing how activities vary in meaningfulness as represented in the activity hierarchy, discussion is warranted regarding certain types of activities that generally are not considered the most meaningful for people with severe disabilities yet still have some relative utility. In an ideal situation, congregate settings would only support consumer involvement in the most therapeutic or meaningful types of activities (i.e., purposeful and age-appropriate activities as represented in the hierarchy). However, as noted previously, consistently involving groups of consumers with severe disabilities in meaningful activities is difficult in many congregate settings. From a practical perspective, when limited resources or other obstacles interfere with an agency's capacity for involving consumers in the most meaningful activities, it is still desirable for consumers to be involved in activities that may be less meaningful but nevertheless have some therapeutic utility or enjoyment value (e.g., purposeful and age-inappropriate activities as illustrated in the hierarchy). In some cases, it is easier for staff to support consumers in the latter types of activities than the former.

Elaboration on the rationale for providing activities of varying degrees of therapeutic value will be presented in subsequent chapter sections. The point here is that agencies should strive to promote consumer involvement in the most meaningful activities but when such involvement is not realistic at times, agencies should still support consumer involvement in activities that are as meaningful as possible. In short, involvement in some activity is usually better than no activity involvement, even if the activity is not the most meaningful.

Purposeful Activities

The most meaningful or therapeutic type of activity for people with severe disabilities in congregate settings is *purposeful* activity. Purposeful activity involves doing something with an apparent purpose, and doing something that would be usual for a person without disabilities to perform. Using leisure materials in the manner the materials are intended to be used by design, working independently, receiving instruction on an habilitative task, and socially interacting with others are common examples of purposeful activities for people with severe disabilities.

Purposeful activities can be either *age-appropriate* or *age-inappropriate*. Activities that are age-appropriate generally are more therapeutic than age-inappropriate activities. An activity in which an individual with severe disabilities is involved is considered age-appropriate if it is an activity in which a nondisabled person who is of the same age group as the individual is likely to participate. Purposeful and age-appropriate activities for adults with severe disabilities, for example, include preparing a snack, playing volleyball, getting dressed, working at a paid job, or talking with another person about what they did over the weekend. These activities are considered age appropriate for adults with severe disabilities because it would be common for adults without disabilities to perform the activities. In contrast, age-inappropriate activities are those that are typically associated with individuals of a younger age group than a respective consumer. Coloring pictures in a coloring book, hugging strangers as a form of greeting, and putting four-piece puzzles of cartoon characters together are examples of purposeful but age-inappropriate activities for adults who have severe disabilities. The latter activities would not normally be observed among the adult population of people without disabilities.

Although considering age-appropriate activities as more therapeutic or beneficial for people with severe disabilities than age-inappropriate activities is well accepted in the professional field, it should also be noted that this issue represents a long-standing controversy among many practitioners. It is beyond the scope of this text to describe the reasons for the controversy over the relative benefits of age-appropriate versus age-inappropriate activities (interested readers are referred to the **Selected Readings** section on **Promoting Meaningful Activity Involvement** for additional information). Suffice it to say that with one notable exception as discussed below, a very considerable amount of research and application has demonstrated the increased benefits of age-appropriate activities relative to age-inappropriate activities.

The exception regarding the greater therapeutic benefits of age-appropriate activities when compared to age-inappropriate activities pertains to leisure situations for people with severe disabilities. Leisure time by definition means that one does what one wants to do within the parameters of accepted social customs and laws. Hence, if a consumer *chooses* to participate in an age-inappropriate activity as a leisure pursuit, then involvement in such an activity is considered acceptable in many human service agencies.

When considering an individual's choice to participate in age-inappropriate leisure activities, special care must be exerted to ensure that such participation is truly the individual's choice. In a number of congregate settings in which there is a predominance of age-inappropriate leisure activities, staff indicate that these activities occur because that is what the consumers prefer. However, on closer examination it is often determined that consumers have not been sufficiently familiarized with other, more age-appropriate options in order to make a meaningful choice to participate in age-appropriate versus age-inappropriate activities. A good rule for ensuring that true choices have been made is to always have some age-appropriate leisure options available. If consumers still choose age-inappropriate activities despite familiarity with, and access to, age-appropriate options, then support staff can be reasonably assured that participation in the former activities truly represents a given consumer's preference.

Participation of people with severe disabilities in *age-inappropriate* activities may be considered acceptable within congregate settings if during leisure times individuals truly choose such activities even though opportunities to participate in *age-appropriate* activities are also immediately available

In regard to the primary focus of this text, participation in purposeful activities—and especially age-appropriate activities—is desirable because such participation contributes to the prevention and treatment of problem behavior. Purposeful activities help consumers learn useful skills that their nondisabled peers typically use on a routine basis. Being skillful in the types of activities in which nondisabled peers participate fosters opportunities for people with disabilities to interact with, and model, individuals who do not have disabilities. Opportunities to model the behavior of nondisabled peers in typical community settings can be an excellent means for people with severe disabilities to learn desirable skills in lieu of learning to display problem behavior.

Participation in purposeful activities also helps people with severe disabilities learn appropriate behaviors that can serve the same purpose as problem behavior and therefore replace the need for problem behavior. In the preceding chapter, it was noted that problem behavior often develops for two primary reasons: to allow an individual to (1) get something the person wants or (2) get out of something the person does not want. As consumers participate in various purposeful activities, they learn more appropriate ways of getting what they want and getting out of what they do not want. To illustrate, if an individual uses aggressive behavior as a means of getting out of an environment with too much ambient noise, learning to operate a CD player to listen to music through headphones may be an appropriate way to reduce or otherwise cover up unwanted noise. Using the CD player, in effect, replaces aggression as a means of escaping a noisy environment.

A final reason for supporting consumer participation in purposeful activities is that such activities contribute to life enjoyment. Having the skills to independently, or with partial support as needed, care for personal needs, work, participate in a variety of leisure activities, and communicate effectively with others forms the basis for a stimulating and enjoyable life. As noted previously, the more enjoyment one experiences on a day-to-day basis, the less likely it is that the individual will engage in challenging behavior.

Engaged Behavior

A relatively common occurrence in many congregate settings for people with severe disabilities, and particularly for people with the most severe disabilities, is that consumers will sometimes be doing something, but what they are doing does not appear to have an apparent purpose (or at least a purpose that is typical of an activity in which nondisabled persons are likely to participate). This type of activity usually involves manipulating various materials but not in the manner the materials are intended to be used by design. An example of this type of apparently nonpurposeful behavior is illustrated by someone stacking puzzle pieces on a table. Puzzle pieces are designed to be fitted together to form a picture rather than being stacked on top of each other. Other examples include turning the pages of a magazine without looking at the magazine, spinning checkers on a table, and shaking a set of headphones.

The type of nonpurposeful activity just illustrated is generally referred to as *engaged* behavior. That is, an individual is engaging the surrounding environment, but not in an apparently purposeful manner. Because engaged behavior does not involve skills or activities that people without disabilities typically display or participate in, and does not involve skills that allow one to function more independently, this type of behavior lacks the benefits of purposeful activity as described earlier. Hence, engaged behavior is considerably less therapeutic or meaningful than purposeful behavior (see the hierarchy of types of activity presented earlier).

Although engaged behavior is considerably less desirable from a therapeutic standpoint than purposeful and age-appropriate or age-inappropriate behavior, engaged behavior can still have some relative benefits for people with severe disabilities in a congregate setting. Because engaged behavior involves manipulation of the surrounding environment, some learning can still occur from this type of activity from an exploratory perspective in much the same way an infant explores the surrounding environment. Additionally, when an individual is busy engaging the surrounding environment, the person is less likely to exhibit problem behavior when compared to participating in no activity.

Engaged behavior is not something that is specifically promoted within congregate settings that desire to provide a therapeutic environment for consumers with severe disabilities. Rather, engaged behavior is more of a by product that occurs when congregate settings are unsuccessful in promoting consistent involvement in purposeful activity. Again though, it can be very difficult to consistently promote purposeful activity among all consumers with severe disabilities in a congregate setting. When participation in purposeful activity is less than optimal, environmental engagement in the manner just described is usually more desirable than the alternative types of activity involvement as described in the following paragraphs.

Nonadaptive and Aggressive/Disruptive Behavior

Whereas each of the types of consumer activity involvement discussed to this point have varying degrees of therapeutic value for people with severe disabilities in congregate settings, there are other types of activities in which individuals can be involved that have no therapeutic utility. The most pervasive type of nontherapeutic activity is *nonadaptive* behavior. Nonadaptive behavior refers to a lack of participation in any type of purposeful or engaged activity, and not displaying aggressive/disruptive or "other" behavior (see later discussion of the latter two types of activities). Repetitive behaviors such as body-rocking or hand-flapping that historically have been referred to as stereotypic behavior represent common examples of nonadaptive behavior. Other examples include pacing around a room with no apparent destination, sitting alone with no other ongoing activity, or simply lying on the floor.

In structured teaching environments such as school classrooms and supported work settings, nonadaptive behavior is often referred to as off-task behavior. That is, consumers are not involved in completing educational or vocational tasks that are expected to be completed in those settings. In residential settings, nonadaptive behavior is most common during typical leisure periods in which consumers are generally expected to be provided with support for participating in leisure activities but for any number of reasons, the support is not sufficient to effectively involve all consumers in the activities.

Frequent occurrence of nonadaptive behavior is a well-established indicator of a nontherapeutic environment within a congregate setting. On a general basis, this type of meaningless activity is often considered *life wasting* among consumers with severe disabilities. Environments in which nonadaptive behavior or life wasting is common are usually characterized by frequent occurrences of problem behavior among one or more consumers.

The other type of consumer activity that has no therapeutic value is *aggressive/disruptive* behavior. Aggressive/disruptive behavior, in which an individual is doing something that is likely to cause harm to a person or the environment, is of course undesired in any environment. Occurrences of aggressive/disruptive behavior require a close look at what is wrong with a consumer's environment, and may necessitate development of an individualized behavior support plan.

Other Behavior

The types of activities just described generally encompass the range of consumer activity involvement that needs to be considered when reviewing the therapeutic quality of a congregate setting for people with severe disabilities. There are, however, other activities in which consumers can also participate. General practice usually combines the latter activities into a generic activity category, simply labeled as *other.* The most common types of "other" activities among consumers with severe disabilities in congregate settings include sleeping, receiving some type of medical attention or participating in a self-care activity by either performing the self-care themselves or receiving assistance from a support staff to complete the self-care (if a support staff person is *teaching* a consumer how to perform the self-care though, then the consumer would be considered to be participating in a therapeutic, purposeful and age-appropriate activity).

As just implied, the "other" activity category generally does not enter significantly into considerations about the therapeutic quality of a congregate setting in terms of the meaningfulness of consumer activity. Consumer time spent in the "other" types of activities is usually rather consistent across respective settings, and simply involves some basic activities of daily living that occur in any congregate setting. These types of activities are mentioned here only because they will be observed at times when reviewing consumer activity involvement, and observers will need to know how to categorize the observations.

Obtaining Formal Measures of Consumer Activity

Once clear indicators of consumer activity involvement have been identified such as by using the activity categorizations just illustrated, the next step within an outcome management approach for increasing therapeutic consumer activities is to implement a means of routinely reviewing the indicators. The indicators must be reviewed on a routine basis in order to obtain objective measures of the degree to which a given setting is effectively promoting consumer involvement in meaningful activities.

One common means through which agency supervisors, clinicians, and evaluators often assess consumer activity involvement is by reviewing consumer activity schedules. Activity schedules specify what activities should be occurring at certain times such as during general leisure time in the late afternoon or early evening. However, although scheduling activities and assigning staff to assist with those activities is often necessary for structuring high levels of consumer activity, a schedule alone is usually not a good indicator of whether consumers *actually participate* in activities. To illustrate, an activity schedule in a group home may indicate that between 4:30 and 5:30, consumers are to be involved in preparing dinner. Direct observations of dinner preparation may reveal though that a staff member is helping one consumer to prepare the meal while three other consumers sit and wait for the meal to be prepared. The latter consumers are not involved in any meaningful activity (i.e., are displaying nonadaptive behavior) and are probably receiving little benefit from the scheduled activity.

A much more accurate indicator of consumer activity than planned schedules involves direct observations in a setting to determine the extent to which consumers actually participate in activities. Without direct observations of the efficacy of supports and services—in this case, representing the degree to which consumers are involved in meaningful activities—there can be no true assurances that agency supports and services are achieving the desired outcomes.

The extent to which consumers participate in meaningful activities can only be accurately determined by directly observing what consumers are doing

Many agencies have formal tools and procedures for observing levels of consumer activity in a given congregate setting. One of the most common approaches that has been used successfully by a number of agencies is outlined in the following chapter sections. The observation system to be described provides an objective and generally straightforward measure of the overall quality and quantity of the activity of people with severe disabilities in congregate situations

Before describing the observation system, it is important to note how the information derived through the process can be used. The system is designed to provide a *global* measure of the quality and quantity of consumer activity in a given congregate setting. Information resulting from the observation process allows evaluative comparisons of the overall level of activity in one setting versus other, similar congregate settings. Information derived from the process also allows a respective agency to evaluate its success in promoting meaningful activity involvement with its consumer group over extended time periods. Most importantly, information derived from the system can alert managers about environments that may be creating likely problem behavior because of consistently low levels of consumer involvement in meaningful activity.

Systematic measures of consumer activity in a given environment using the system to be described can also be useful to authors of behavior support plans. If objective measures indicate that consumers are not participating in meaningful activities very often, authors of support plans should be aware that the likelihood of effectively treating problem behavior is quite low. Having documentation of the level of meaningful activity in a respective environment may help clinicians charged with developing support plans to convince supervisors and other relevant personnel that the environment warrants improvement prior to developing a treatment plan for an individual consumer. As indicated in earlier chapters, the initial focus of an intervention for a consumer's challenging behavior should be an evaluation of the adequacy of the consumer's surrounding environment, and the degree of involvement in meaningful activities should be a primary focus of the evaluation.

It should be emphasized that the observation system to be described is meant to evaluate an environment for a *group* of consumers (e.g., a group of residents in a group home, a group of students in a classroom). The system is not designed to gauge the therapeutic quality of activities for an individual consumer. The activity definitions described earlier that constitute the indices of environmental quality to be observed do not take into consideration an individual consumer's treatment goals and preferred activities, which would be necessary components of a system for evaluating environmental quality for a given individual. Also, the system focuses on activities of all consumers in a respective group, such that a detailed analysis of activity involvement for one particular consumer is not provided.

Conducting Observations

Objectively and accurately observing indices of environmental quality is facilitated if the observations are completed using a prepared observation form. A prototypical observation form developed specifically for observing activity involvement among people with severe disabilities in congregate settings is represented in the following **Group Activity Observation Form**.

To use the **Group Activity Observation Form**, the observer (e.g., staff supervisor, author of a behavior support plan) first completes the descriptive information at the top of the form including the date, time, setting in which the observation will occur, and who is conducting the observation. Next, the observer enters the setting where the observation is to be conducted and lists each of the consumers present in the spaces provided on the left side of the form, with one consumer identified per space. Consumers do not need to be identified by name—again, the purpose of this observation system is to obtain information about the level of meaningful activity for the entire *group* of consumers. The identification of consumers can be conducted simply by using, for example, distinctive features of each consumer's clothing.

Once the descriptive information is provided on the **Group Activity Observation Form**, the first consumer listed on the form is then observed very briefly (three to five seconds), and what the consumer is doing when *first* observed is determined using the categories of activities described earlier. That is, the consumer's observed activity should be recorded as purposeful and age-appropriate, purposeful and age-inappropriate, engaged, nonadapative, aggressive/disruptive or other. The type of activity observed is noted by marking a slash ("/") through the symbol for the corresponding activity category in the column directly to the right of the identified consumer. Only one category of activity should be marked when a consumer is observed. The remaining consumers are then observed one after another in sequence as they are listed on the observation form. Approximately 10 seconds should be allowed between observations of each consumer.

The observation process should continue until at least 10 samples of consumer activity are obtained in a given environment. If there are less than 10 consumers in the environment, individual consumers can be observed up to three times in order to obtain at least 10 samples. The second and third columns of activity symbols on the observation form are used when necessary for repeated observations of an individual consumer in order to obtain the 10 samples. Figure 4-3 illustrates a completed **Group Activity Observation Form**.

GROUP ACTIVITY OBSERVATION FORM

Setting: ______________________________

Date: __________ Time: __________ Monitor: __________

ACTIVITY CODES	
Purposeful/Age Appropriate: PA	Nonadaptive: N
Purposeful/Age Inappropriate: PI	Aggressive/Disruptive: AD
Engaged: E	Other: O

Individual	Activity		
1. ________	PA PI E N AD O	PA PI E N AD O	PA PI E N AD O
2. ________	PA PI E N AD O	PA PI E N AD O	PA PI E N AD O
3. ________	PA PI E N AD O	PA PI E N AD O	PA PI E N AD O
4. ________	PA PI E N AD O	PA PI E N AD O	PA PI E N AD O
5. ________	PA PI E N AD O	PA PI E N AD O	PA PI E N AD O
6. ________	PA PI E N AD O	PA PI E N AD O	PA PI E N AD O
7. ________	PA PI E N AD O	PA PI E N AD O	PA PI E N AD O
8. ________	PA PI E N AD O	PA PI E N AD O	PA PI E N AD O
9. ________	PA PI E N AD O	PA PI E N AD O	PA PI E N AD O
10. ________	PA PI E N AD O	PA PI E N AD O	PA PI E N AD O

DATA SUMMARY

Total of: PA____ PI____ E____ N____ AD____ O____

Total number of intervals observed: _____

% occurrence: PA___ PI___ E___ N___ AD___ O___

Figure 4-2: Group Activity Observation Form for observing activity involvement of people with severe disabilities in congregate settings.

GROUP ACTIVITY OBSERVATION FORM

Setting: Main Street Work Center

Date: 8-17 Time: 9:45 Monitor: Jackson

ACTIVITY CODES

Purposeful/Age Appropriate: PA	Nonadaptive: N
Purposeful/Age Inappropriate: PI	Aggressive/Disruptive: AD
Engaged: E	Other: O

Individual	Activity		
1. White shirt	PA PI E N AD O	PA PI E N AD O	PA PI E N AD O
2. Cap	PA PI E N AD O	PA PI E N AD O	PA PI E N AD O
3. Red blouse	PA PI E N AD O	PA PI E N AD O	PA PI E N AD O
4. Blue shirt	PA PI E N AD O	PA PI E N AD O	PA PI E N AD O
5. Green dress	PA PI E N AD O	PA PI E N AD O	PA PI E N AD O
6. Black shirt	PA PI E N AD O	PA PI E N AD O	PA PI E N AD O
7. Striped shirt	PA PI E N AD O	PA PI E N AD O	PA PI E N AD O
8. T-shirt	PA PI E N AD O	PA PI E N AD O	PA PI E N AD O
9. NY cap	PA PI E N AD O	PA PI E N AD O	PA PI E N AD O
10. Grey dress	PA PI E N AD O	PA PI E N AD O	PA PI E N AD O

DATA SUMMARY

Total of: PA 10 PI 5 E___ N 5 AD___ O___

Total number of intervals observed: ____

% occurrence: PA 50 PI 25 E___ N 25 AD___ O___

Figure 4-3: Sample of a completed *Group Activity Observation Form.*

Summarizing Results of Observations

Once the observation is completed, the number of samples obtained for each category of activity are counted. The percentage of samples for which each activity category was observed is then calculated by dividing the number of samples in each activity category by the total number of samples obtained, and multiplying by 100%. The completed **Group Activity Observation Form** just illustrated reflects how the recordings are summarized.

Note that on the observation form completed for Main Street Work Center on August 17, there were 20 samples of activities observed across all consumers. During 10 of the samples (50%) the consumers were involved in an age-appropriate, purposeful activity. In five of the samples (25%) the consumers were observed doing something that was purposeful, but age-inappropriate. In the remaining five samples (25%), consumers were involved in nonadaptive behavior.

A concise yet informative summary of the quality and quantity of consumer activity in a given congregate setting can be provided by graphing the percentages of purposeful activities and nonadaptive activities over several observation sessions. The following graph illustrates how results from multiple observations in an environment can be presented for quick review. The graph shows that the activities at Main Street Work Center were observed once each week during June, July and August. The percentage of purposeful and nonadaptive behavior resulting from each observation is plotted on the graph. For example, during the third week in August, as reflected on the previously illustrated, completed **Group Activity Observation Form** on August 17, purposeful behavior was at 75% (i.e., 50% purposeful age-appropriate plus 25% purposeful, age-inappropriate) and nonadaptive behavior was at 25%.

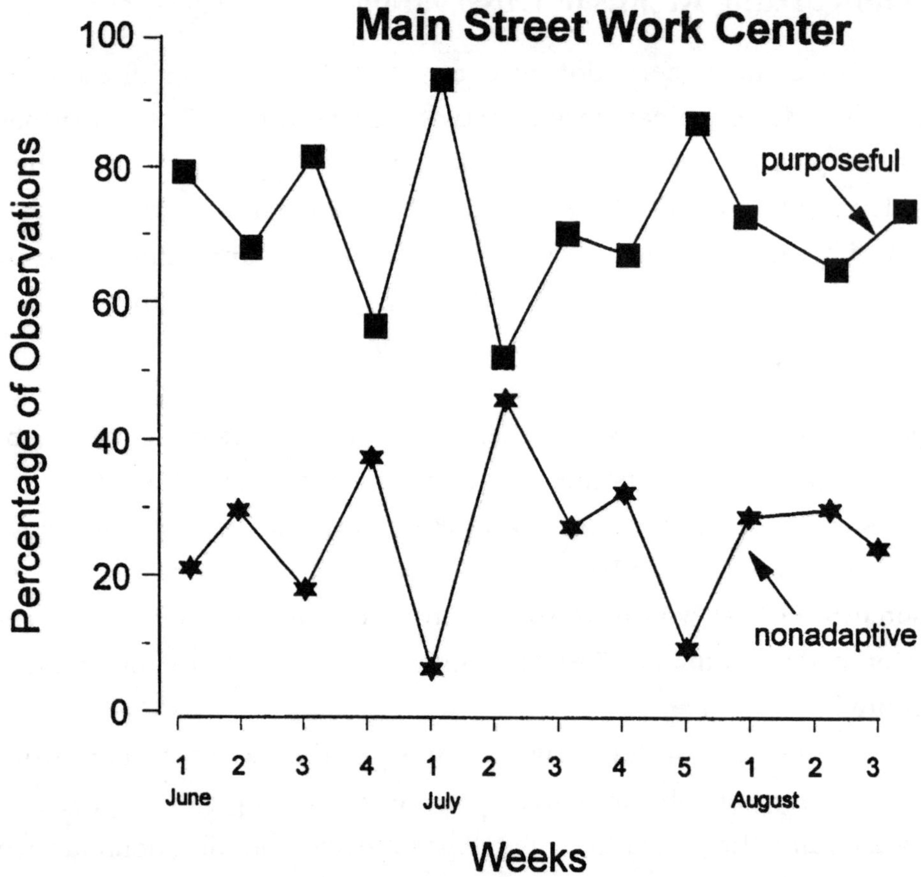

Figure 4-4: Percentage of observations with purposeful and nonadaptive activity among people with severe disabilities from June through the third week in August at Main Street Work Center.

Evaluating and Interpreting Measures of Consumer Activity

Once several observations in an environment have produced a pattern of activity like the one just illustrated, decisions must be made as to whether improvements are needed regarding consumer involvement in therapeutic activities. To make such decisions, an agency must first specify an acceptable level of activity for a given setting (e.g., a particular residential unit, work enclave, adult education or activity classroom). When a respective environment falls below the desired level during several observations, action should then be taken to improve the frequency or type of activity.

What constitutes an acceptable level of consumer activity will vary depending on the type of setting and the characteristics of consumers in the environment. It is generally reasonable to expect that a day treatment setting in which the staff-to-consumer ratio is approximately 1:4 on average, for example, would have a higher level of meaningful activity than a residential program in which the staff-to-consumer ratio is approximately 1:6. Residential settings for people with severe multiple disabilities in which each consumer requires individual assistance from a staff member to participate in leisure activities would be expected to have a lower activity level on average than a setting in which consumers have independent or near independent leisure skills.

To assist with identifying satisfactory levels of activity, the following figure shows the results of an observational, normative sampling of activity patterns in two types of environments. Both environments represent day treatment programs for adults with severe disabilities who are ambulatory. The first bar graph on the figure (left side of figure) represents community-based programs such as adult education or activity classrooms and sheltered workshops, and the second bar graph (right side of figure) represents day programs operated by state institutions. The activity levels presented in the figure are based on observations in more than 100 settings across the United States.

By comparing the activity pattern obtained in a respective day treatment setting to normative averages like those depicted in the figure, agency personnel can determine if the consumer activity in their own setting is better or worse than the average activity pattern in similar settings. To illustrate, consider the example noted earlier with the Main Street Work Center in which the level of purposeful activity over serveral months averaged close to 70%. Such an activity level compares favorably with the normative averages from both community-based and facility-based day treatment programs, in which the average level of adaptive behavior is approximately 50%.

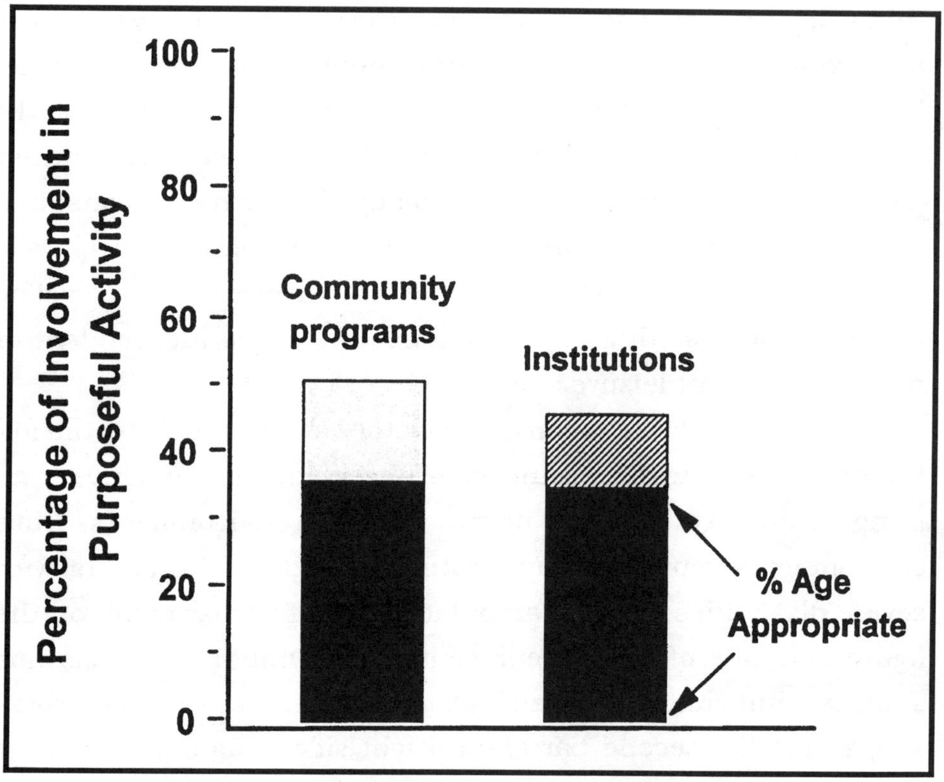

Figure 4-5: Results of normative observations of individuals with severe disabilities (ambulatory) in congregate day treatment settings around the United States, showing the average amount of observed time involved in purposeful activity, and the portion of purposeful activity that was age appropriate. Drawn from Reid, D.H., Parsons, M.B., & Green, C.W. (2001). Evaluating the functional utility of congregate day treatment activities for adults with severe disabilities. *American Journal on Mental Retardation, 106,* 460-469.

Conducting Informal Measures of Activity Involvement

Because of the difficulties inherent in promoting meaningful activity involvement among people with severe disabilities in congregate settings, it is generally desirable to use a formal system such as the process just described to routinely evaluate activity involvement. It also can be beneficial to supplement a formal system with more informal monitoring procedures for reviewing activity involvement. Informal evaluative approaches involving brief observations of consumer activity offer several benefits relative to the more formal systems. The latter procedures can be especially helpful for authors of behavior support plans who may not have control over, or be involved in, formal evaluative processes concerning routine consumer activities.

A primary benefit of informal means of observing and evaluating consumer activity involvement is that the procedures can be conducted in a very efficient manner. Additionally, whereas formal monitoring systems usually occur on a preplanned, scheduled basis in order to systematically assess a variety of situations across different time periods, informal monitoring procedures can be completed at essentially any time with no prior preparation. Supervisors and authors of behavior support plans can incorporate informal monitoring of consumer activities within many of their other routine duties whenever they are present in a respective setting.

An informal approach to observing and evaluating consumer activity involvement can be conducted using the categories of activities described earlier. The process involves a supervisor or clinician quickly determining the percentage of consumers who are involved in purposeful activities each time the person enters the setting of concern. To illustrate, a psychologist could quickly calculate the percentage of consumers who are doing something purposeful in a group home each time the psychologist visits the home. The psychologist simply counts how many consumers are present in a specific area (e.g., living room), then counts the number of consumers involved in purposeful activities and determines or estimates the percentage of the latter consumers out of all consumers present. By repeating this quick observation process whenever the psychologist visits the home, the psychologist can stay consistently aware of the general activity pattern in the home. Using the quick method of observation just described, agency supervisors and clinical personnel can readily pinpoint troublesome times of day or locations for which consumer involvement in activities warrants improvement. Subsequently, efforts can be directed to increasing activity participation during those situations. As problematic situations are improved, the improvements should be reflected in the results of the agency's more formal observation system for reviewing consumer activity involvement.

Increasing Consumer Involvement in Therapeutic Activity

When indicators of consumer activity involvement are unsatisfactory, whether based on formal or informal review procedures, supervisors must determine how to improve consumer activity. It is beyond the scope of this text to describe in-depth the various means of increasing consumer involvement in purposeful activities (again, see **Promoting Meaningful Activity Involvement** section of the **Selected Readings**). However, two variables warrant mention that are particularly important for ensuring a therapeutic level of purposeful activity among people with severe disabilities in congregate settings. These variables are the *availability of materials* and the *frequency of staffs' teaching interactions.*

The degree to which staff make leisure and habilitative materials readily accessible to consumers and then support consumer use of the materials through effective teaching interactions has a major impact on consumer activity involvement. Hence, how staff perform these aspects of their jobs warrants attention when considering ways to increase or maintain purposeful activity. The following **Group Activity Process Observation Form** illustrates a means through which a number of agencies effectively evaluate and promote staffs' proficiency in maintaining material availability and support consumer use of the materials. The **Group Activity Process Observation Form** is designed to diagnose problems in the *process* of promoting activity involvement among consumers and subsequently, to indicate what needs to occur to improve such involvement.

Group Activity Process Observation Form

Setting: ________________ Date: ______ Time: _____ Monitor: __________

Recording Section

Number of consumers present at the beginning of the observation: _____

Number of consumers with materials within arm's reach: _____

Number of consumers receiving a teaching interaction from staff: _____

Number of consumer present at the end of the observation: _____

Summarization Section

Average number of consumers present: _____

Percentage of consumers with materials within arm's reach: _____

Percentage of consumers receiving a teaching interaction: _____

Figure 4-6: *Group Activity Process Observation Form* for monitoring the process of promoting purposeful activity involvement among people with severe disabilities in congregate settings.

To use the **Group Activity Process Observation Form**, the identifying information at the top of the form should be completed just before entering the environment where the observation is to occur. Upon entering the environment, four pieces of information are recorded. First, the number of consumers present in the environment at the beginning of the observation is recorded. Second, the number of consumers who have ready access to a leisure or work material is counted. Ready access to materials is defined as a consumer having a leisure or work material within arm's reach. Third, all staff and consumers are simultaneously observed for two minutes and the number of consumers who receive a teaching interaction is recorded. Teaching interactions are defined as prompting an individual to participate in an activity by using the available materials or praising (reinforcing) an individual for participating in the activity. For example, an interaction consisting of a staff member physically guiding a consumer to shoot a basketball would be counted as a teaching interaction because the staff member is prompting a purposeful activity (in this case, a purposeful leisure activity). Likewise, a staff member praising a consumer's actions when the consumer turns on the oven to bake a cake represents a teaching interaction, because baking a cake represents a purposeful activity. Finally, the fourth step of the observation process involves counting the number of consumers present in the environment at the end of the observation. The entire observation process generally requires no more than three to four minutes to complete.

The section at the bottom of the **Group Activity Process Observation Form** indicates how the data obtained during the observation should be summarized. The average number of consumers in the environment is obtained by summing the number of consumers present at the beginning and end of the observation session and dividing by two. The two numbers are averaged together because some consumers may enter or leave the room during the observation, and the average presents a more accurate indication of the number of consumers present throughout the observation than the number present at the beginning or end of the observation. Next, the percentage of consumers with materials within arms' reach is obtained by dividing the number of consumers who were observed with materials within arm's reach by the average number of consumers present in the environment and multiplying the result by 100%. The same calculation process is used for determining the percentage of consumers who received a teaching interaction. The following illustration of a completed **Group Activity Process Observation Form** shows how the results of an observation conducted with the form are summarized.

Group Activity Process Observation Form

Setting: Asheville St. Home Date: 8/18 Time: 6:00 Monitor: BB

Recording Section

Number of consumers present at the beginning of the observation: 4

Number of consumers with materials within arm's reach: 4

Number of consumers receiving a teaching interaction from staff: 1

Number of consumer present at the end of the observation: 6

Summarization Section

Average number of consumers present: 5

Percentage of consumers with materials within arm's reach: 4/5 = 80%

Percentage of consumers receiving a teaching interaction: 1/5 = 20%

Figure 4-7: Sample completed *Group Activity Process Observation Form.*

Results of applied research with the **Group Activity Process Observation Form** have indicated that when the percentage of consumers who have materials within arm's reach and the percentage of consumers who receive a teaching interaction during an observation are both 80% or more, consumer activity involvement is likely to be at a therapeutic level. If observations indicate that the percentage of consumers who have materials within arm's reach or receive a teaching interaction is less than 80%, supervisory action is usually needed to improve one or both of these situations.

Ensuring the Availability of Materials

A brief tour in many congregate residential settings for people with severe disabilities often reveals staff attempting to involve groups of consumers in activities using only a few materials. In some sheltered work settings, a similar situation is frequently observed in that work materials are not available due to an inconsistent supply of work from contracting agencies. In these types of situations, where there are few materials to support consumer involvement in activities, observations will almost invariably reveal low levels of consumer activity. Although having an abundance of leisure or work materials will not ensure that consumers will be involved in meaningful activities, a lack of sufficient materials will almost always guarantee that consumers will not be involved in meaningful activities very often.

One rather straightforward means of ensuring materials are accessible to consumers is to include the duty of managing materials within the daily work assignments of respective staff. Each day, someone should have the designated responsibility of ensuring that materials are available at appropriate times, broken materials are repaired or replaced in a timely fashion, and a ready supply of batteries is on hand for materials that require batteries for operation. Simply making this type of material manager assignment, and effectively supervising staff in fulfilling the assignment (see **Chapters**

10 and **11**), can go a long way toward ensuring material availability and consumer activity involvement.

A prerequisite for promoting frequent involvement of people with severe disabilities in meaningful activities in congregate settings is consistent availability of leisure and habilitative materials

Utilize Group Teaching Techniques

If observations with the **Group Activity Process Observation Form** frequently reveal that less than 80% of consumers are receiving teaching interactions from staff concerning use of available materials (i.e., staff are not consistently prompting or praising consumer use of the materials), supervisors should focus their attention on increasing staffs' teaching interactions. In order to ensure staff interact with consumers sufficiently to promote activity involvement, several supervisory actions typically must be considered. These actions coincide with an outcome management approach to staff supervision.

The desired outcome in the situation described here is that staff engage in frequent teaching interactions and consumers frequently interact with available materials as a means of participating in purposeful activity. To attain the outcome, supervisors must make sure staff have been adequately trained in how to prompt and reinforce consumer use of the materials (see **Chapter 7** for an in-depth discussion of effective staff training procedures). Additionally, it is important that staff be trained in how to distribute their interactions among all consumers present in the setting.

Distribution of teaching interactions across all consumers is a critical variable affecting consumer activity involvement in group situations when there are more consumers than staff. There is often a tendency for staff to interact with certain individuals in a given group more than with other individuals. Such a process usually means that the latter individuals will not be participating in purposeful activities. Staff should be instructed in how to frequently rotate their attention every few minutes or so across different individuals. In this manner, no consumer will go for long periods of time without receiving support for participating in meaningful activities.

In addition to ensuring that all consumers receive support to interact with materials through effective prompting and reinforcing by staff, consumer activity involvement can be enhanced if staff provide consumers with frequent choices of materials with which to interact. When staff provide frequent material choices for consumers, the individuals are more likely to access materials and activities that they prefer relative to situations in which staff simply provide materials without regard for individual preferences. Having access to preferred materials makes it more likely that consumers will use the materials as well as enjoy their use. As indicated in preceding chapters, when individuals with severe disabilities enjoy what they are doing, there is little likelihood of problem behavior occurring.

Once support staff have been trained in how to distribute their interactions by rotating across consumers as well as how to provide choices, prompt and reinforce use of materials, then the other component steps of outcome management can be implemented. The latter procedures, which are designed to support or correct staffs' teaching interactions with consumers as necessary, are discussed in detail in **Chapters 10** and **11**.

Special Considerations for Authors of Behavior Support Plans

Preceding chapter sections provided several suggestions that are particularly relevant for clinicians and other personnel who develop behavior support plans for challenging behavior. Most notably, authors of plans should attend to indices of consumer activity involvement. When there is a low level of involvement in purposeful activities and high levels of nonadaptive behavior, authors should work with agency management and supervisors to improve meaningful activity involvement. When purposeful activity involvement is high, authors should make special attempts to recognize staff and supervisors who are responsible for promoting meaningful activity.

Attention directed to consumer activity involvement should occur *before* a clinician attempts to develop an individualized support plan for a respective consumer's problem behavior. As noted repeatedly, problem behavior can rarely be treated in a problematic environment, and lack of frequent involvement in purposeful activity is usually indicative of a problematic environment. Relatedly, when a consumer displays challenging behavior within an environment that is relatively void of meaningful activity options, often the consumer's behavior is not really the problem; the environment is the problem.

To help agencies providing services in congregate settings, authors of support plans should advocate for agency management to employ regular means of evaluating and responding to objective measures of consumer activity involvement. The observation system and corresponding norms for purposeful activity involvement presented in this chapter represents one means of accurately monitoring and evaluating activity involvement for groups of consumers that has proven useful in many congregate settings. However, treatment plan authors should always conduct their own, informal measures of consumer activity involvement as also illustrated earlier. Frequent observations of what consumers are doing can be of considerable utility for assessing what should be done to prevent and treat challenging behavior.

CHAPTER 5

Teaching Meaningful Skills: A Critical But Under-Emphasized Component for Preventing and Treating Challenging Behavior

The importance of supporting individuals with severe disabilities in purposeful leisure and social activities was heavily stressed in the preceding chapter. Frequent involvement in meaningful activities as described in **Chapter 4** represents a well-established indicator of a therapeutic environment. When an agency consistently involves its consumers in meaningful activities, and particularly activities that consumers find enjoyable, the agency is taking a major step toward preventing the occurrence of challenging behavior.

If people with severe disabilities are to be involved in meaningful activities, they must have the skills to functionally participate in the activities. In turn, for individuals with severe disabilities to learn meaningful or functional skills, support staff must help teach those skills to individual consumers. Consistent provision of teaching services that focus on functional skill development is another primary indicator of a therapeutic environment for people with severe disabilities.

Providing quality teaching services also has a major impact on the prevention and treatment of challenging behavior. The significance of teaching programs in this respect is due primarily to the reasons challenging behavior often occurs. As indicated in previous chapters, a major reason why people with severe disabilities display challenging behavior is that they have not learned more appropriate ways of expressing their wants and needs. Instead, aggression, self-injury, and other types of problem behavior are used to indicate to support personnel that they do or do not want to do something. If individuals are taught skills that allow them to achieve the function that their problem behavior typically achieves, then they have little need for problem behavior. Hence, the more useful skills staff can teach to consumers with severe disabilities, the less likely it becomes that consumers will use challenging behavior to meet their needs.

Teaching functional and meaningful skills to individuals who have severe disabilities also decreases the likelihood of challenging behavior in more general ways. In particular, the more functional skills one acquires, the more independent the person becomes. Increased independence by definition means people acquire more control over their lives. For consumers with severe disabilities, increased independence and control means that they do more things for themselves relative to support staff doing things for them. As people gain control over their lives in this manner, the more enjoyable their lives become. People usually prefer to meet their needs themselves in contrast to being dependent on others to meet their needs. As noted repeatedly already, the more enjoyable one's life, the less likely it is that challenging behavior will be displayed.

In short, teaching functional skills to people who have severe disabilities helps them to live more independently and enjoyably, as well as to live without the numerous obstacles and problems associated with challenging behavior. Recognition of the critical importance of teaching functional skills has resulted in an immense amount of research and application on how to teach individuals who have severe disabilities. Literally hundreds of applied research articles and texts describe a very effective technology of teaching for people who have severe disabilities.

As more functional skills are taught to individuals with severe disabilities, the less likely it becomes that challenging behavior will occur

Although considerable attention has been directed to methods of teaching people with severe disabilities, much less attention has focused on *what* should be taught. From the perspective of preventing and treating challenging behavior, attention usually needs to be directed to the types of skills that represent the focus of teaching programs in congregate settings. Attention to what is taught is usually needed because despite the importance of functional skill development on the prevention and treatment of challenging behavior, this aspect of agency supports and services is often overlooked for consumers who display problem behavior. Reasons for the relative lack of attention in this regard will be illustrated later. On a more basic level, concern over teaching services is often warranted because teaching programs that do exist in congregate settings frequently do not address skills that are very meaningful.

Concern over lack of meaningful teaching services is exemplified in the observational data presented in **Chapter 4**. Observations on which the normative data presented in **Chapter 4** are based have demonstrated that in a number of day treatment settings such as sheltered workshops and adult activity programs, there is minimal or no involvement of consumers in activities that are likely to teach meaningful skills. Similar concerns exist with a number of school classrooms serving students with severe disabilities; students are often observed being taught skills that are not purposeful or that are purposeful only for children who are much younger than the students.

There are numerous reasons why teaching programs for people with severe disabilities in congregate settings focus on nonfunctional or nonmeaningful skills. However, essentially all of the reasons can be resolved if staff follow several well-established guidelines when determining what to teach to consumers with whom they work. The purpose of this chapter is to review those guidelines. The intent is to help establish meaningful teaching programs for people with severe disabilities, and to replace existing programs that focus on nonfunctional skills with programs that address more meaningful and functional skills. If the guidelines to be presented are adhered to, then agency consumers are much more likely to learn skills that enable them to live more independently and enjoyably. Most relevant for the focus of this text, adherence to the guidelines will make it less likely that challenging behavior will occur, and will enhance the effectiveness of support plans for challenging behavior that does occur.

Guidelines for Determining Functional Skills for Teaching Programs

Before presenting guidelines for determining functional or meaningful skills to teach to people with severe disabilities, the criterion for purposeful activities as described in the preceding chapter warrants review. Purposeful activities—which inherently involve functional or meaningful skills—were described in **Chapter 4** as activities in which it would be usual for people without disabilities to participate. It was further noted that the most therapeutic types of purposeful activities in congregate settings involve activities in which people without disabilities typically participate who are of the same age group as a respective agency's consumers.

This definition of purposeful activities is most useful when considering leisure and general social pursuits of people with severe disabilities. The definition is also relevant for other types of activities such as daily living or personal care routines, communicative interactions, and vocational endeavors. However, for the latter types of activities, several more specific guidelines can facilitate the determination of functional versus nonfunctional skills to teach to individuals with severe disabilities.

Guideline #1: Functional Skills Involve Activities That Someone Else Would Have to Do for an Individual If the Individual Could Not Do the Activities

Identifying meaningful skills to teach to a consumer based on whether the skills would be performed for the consumer if the consumer could not do the skills is the longest-standing criterion for selecting functional skills. This guideline is particularly relevant for determining useful self-help skills to teach to people with severe disabilities. For example, if an individual does not have the skills to button his shirt, then it would be functional for someone to teach him to button his shirt because otherwise, a support staff would have to button his shirt for him. Teaching an individual how to brush her hair would likewise be functional because if she did not brush her hair, a support person would have to brush her hair for her. In contrast, teaching someone to identify and point to buttons on people's clothing in magazine pictures or to brush a doll's hair would not be functional skills to teach. In the latter cases, no one would perform the skills (i.e., point to pictures of buttons or brush a doll's hair) for the individual if the person could not do those things.

A good way to apply this guideline for selecting functional skills is to consider the daily routine of an individual consumer, and identify everything that support staff do for the consumer during the routine. Those things that support staff routinely do for the consumer, ranging from dressing the individual to preparing the individual's food, represent sets of skills that would be functional to teach the consumer to perform.

Teaching individuals who have severe disabilities to perform self-help types of skills has long been recognized as a meaningful goal of teaching programs. Clearly, the more individuals can take care of their personal needs themselves, the more independently they can lead their lives. Teaching people with severe disabilities to perform their own self-help activities also has a direct bearing on the likelihood of challenging behavior occurring. Whenever support staff must perform a self-care activity for an individual, the staff must have close physical contact with the individual and frequently, physically guide the person through necessary movements to complete the activity. At times, people like physical contact and guidance from other persons. At other times though, people do not like such contact and guidance. In some situations, individuals do not mind contact and guidance from certain support staff but dislike the contact and guidance from other staff. When consumers do not like such actions, problem behavior may result in an attempt by consumers to escape or avoid the undesired activity. By teaching consumers to perform their own self-care routines, and thereby eliminate the need for staff to physically contact the consumers in order to complete the self-care activity, certain types of challenging behavior can be prevented.

Another reason the development of independent self-care skills can reduce the likelihood of challenging behavior pertains to personal preferences. Most people prefer to take care of their personal needs, such as combing their hair, putting on their own make-up, and selecting the clothes they will wear for the day. When support staff perform these duties for consumers because the individuals cannot perform the necessary skills, self-care activities can become less pleasant for the consumers relative to them performing the skills in the manner they prefer. Unpleasant activities are much more likely to be accompanied by challenging behavior than pleasant activities.

As individuals with severe disabilities learn skills to perform self-help routines for themselves, then problem behavior associated with staff performing those duties for the individuals is eliminated

Guideline #2: The More Frequently a Person is Likely to Perform a Skill, the More Functional the Skill is to Teach

A second useful guideline for determining functional skills to teach is based on how often the skills are likely to be needed or used by an individual. Generally, the more frequently a skill is used, the more functional it is to teach. To illustrate, a social skill that is usually very functional to teach a consumer is how to greet someone such as a work colleague or support staff when the consumer first sees the person during the day. Opportunities to greet people typically occur multiple times during the day. In contrast, a social skill such as how to perform a certain dance step is not likely to be needed on a daily or even weekly basis. Hence, it is usually more useful to spend time teaching a consumer how to greet people than spending the time teaching how to dance.

In the situation just illustrated, it should not be assumed that teaching how to dance would never be useful or functional. Rather, the issue is that social skills that can be used frequently such as greeting others generally represent more functional goals of teaching services than social skills that are used infrequently. Once individuals learn social skills that they can use often, then the focus of teaching can shift to social skills that are needed less often (but still needed).

Guideline #3: Skills for Which a Person Can Be Paid to Perform as Part of a Job Are Functional Skills to Teach

A third guideline for selecting functional skills to teach pertains to vocational endeavors. Specifically, those skills for which someone can be paid to perform as part of a job represent functional skills to teach. This guideline is most relevant for adults with severe disabilities, but also pertains to adolescents in terms of acquiring the skills to enter the work force and obtain a part- or full-time job once they finish school.

In concept, the notion that skills for which people can be paid to perform as part of a job represent functional skills to teach is straightforward. The benefits of assisting people with severe disabilities in obtaining real jobs have become very apparent through advances made in supported employment. In order to obtain and maintain gainful employment though, individuals must have the skills to perform the necessary work either on their own or with staff support. Nonetheless, observations in many sheltered workshops and adult activity centers have shown that large numbers of adults with severe disabilities spend time learning or doing tasks under the guise of vocational services with no likelihood of earning an income.

In many adult day programs, consumers are involved in nonpaid activities with the expressed purpose of helping the consumers learn skills that they could later apply in paid work situations. Common activities of this nature include sorting beads by color, putting plastic nuts on plastic bolts, and counting and sorting piles of popsicle sticks. The intent is that consumers will learn sorting skills, assembly skills, counting skills, etc., that could later be applied to real job situations. Despite such an intent, these types of activities do not meet the criterion for teaching functional vocational skills. The activities usually amount to busy work at best, and at worst, life wasting.

Nonpaid activities such as those just illustrated that are common in many vocational programs for people with severe disabilities generally have no true utility for two reasons. First, once people begin these types of "prevocational" preparation activities, frequently they never have subsequent opportunities to obtain paid jobs. The consumers are considered to be receiving vocational services and as such, are viewed as having their vocational needs met. Second, whatever skills the consumers learn in these activities typically have little or no bearing on the skills they need to fulfill a job responsibility. In some cases, job opportunities that may arise have no relationship to what the consumers spend their time doing in the prevocational setting, such that they have to learn other skills that can be used on the job. In other cases, skills such as sorting or counting may be relevant to a job, but consumers have difficulty generalizing their skills from the prevocational setting to the job.

Problems in generalizing skills from nonpaid day treatment activities to real job situations often occur because the materials used in the former settings are very different from the materials used on the job. For example, a consumer may learn to sort beads by color in a classroom, but then experience difficulty when expected to sort manual pages or other paper products as part of a clerical job. The latter materials are too different from the former materials for the consumer to be able to transfer sorting skills across the two different situations.

To avoid problems with skill generalization as just exemplified, programs designed to teach vocational skills should involve the same materials that a consumer would use during a regular job. Again, from a vocational perspective, a skill is functional to teach only if the skill is one for which a person could be paid to perform as part of a regular job. If the materials used in the teaching program are not the same materials that would be used on the job, then the person would not be paid to do that activity as part of a real job.

In addition to the issues noted to this point regarding nonpaid activities in adult day programs, there is a concern with these types of services that often is raised in regard to the impact on challenging behavior among consumers attending the programs. Many sheltered workshops and adult activity programs have been criticized for involving people with severe disabilities in highly repetitive activities that involve doing the same thing (e.g., sorting, putting nuts on bolts) hour after hour, day after day, etc. Such activities frequently are viewed as requiring consumers to participate in dull, monotonous work that has little meaning for the consumers. The emphasis on repetitive, monotonous work is likewise considered to result in serious problem behavior among many consumers in an attempt to avoid the undesired work. Challenging behavior can also occur in the form of consumers tantruming, aggressing, or otherwise refusing to leave their residence in the morning in an attempt to avoid having to go to the day program.

The concern just noted regarding many day program activities is justified in a number of cases. Some consumers do find repetitive types of activities unattractive, and with no other recourse available, use problem behavior in an attempt to avoid doing the work. However, the concern is not warranted in its entirety for other consumers. There are some types of jobs that involve highly repetitive activities for which individuals can earn relatively decent wages. There are also some individuals with severe disabilities who prefer to work on repetitive duties, just like some workers without disabilities prefer this type of work.

The point of concern here is that the specific type of work is not as important as the activity preferences of individual workers. Support staff and executive personnel in day programs should not be the ones who decide what represents preferred versus nonpreferred work. Rather, that decision should be made based on the preferences of individual workers.

There is a considerable body or applied research that demonstrates how to assess work preferences among people with severe disabilities (see **Determining Consumer Activity Preferences** in the **Selected Readings**). As much as possible, work assignments should be based on the assessed preferences of each worker. It is well established that individuals with severe disabilities work harder on tasks that they prefer relative to tasks that they do not prefer. Similarly, when workers have opportunities to choose what to work on out of several alternatives, they will usually work harder relative to being told what to work on by support staff. By providing choices of work tasks and access to work preferences, day programs can enhance the work performance and productivity of workers with severe disabilities.

Providing choices of work tasks and access to work preferences can also have a major impact on the prevention and treatment of challenging behavior. When individuals are working diligently—due at least in part to having opportunities to work on preferred tasks—they are not likely to engage in problem behavior. Working on a task and engaging in problem behavior are simply incompatible activities. Additionally, when individuals are doing things that they tend to enjoy, the likelihood of problem behavior is decreased relative to doing things that are disliked.

By providing individuals with choices of work tasks and access to preferred work, not only is work performance and productivity enhanced, the likelihood of problem behavior is decreased

To be able to match consumer preferences with assigned work tasks, it is helpful if congregate settings that provide vocationally related services offer a variety of work options. Generally, the highest quality day programs of a congregate nature provide a wide range of activities. Such activities include, for example, various work tasks that are completed at a work table (which are beneficial for workers who prefer to sit and work) as well as more active tasks such as those performed by mobile work crews (for workers who prefer to be physically active). Tasks that involve social interactions with others (for workers who like social attention) as well as tasks that can be performed in a solitary manner (for workers who prefer to work alone) also are usually provided. Basically, the more work options that exist, the greater the likelihood that work assignments for respective workers can be selected based on the work preferences of the workers.

Guideline # 4: Skills That Allow a Person to Get Something Wanted Or Get Out Something Unwanted Without Problem Behavior Are Functional Skills to Teach

The final guideline regarding identification of functional skills to teach relates most directly to the prevention and treatment of challenging behavior. This guideline involves skills that are functional because the skills allow a person to get something wanted or to get out of something unwanted without the need for challenging behavior. In most cases, these types of functional skills involve teaching individuals appropriate means of communicating what they want and do not want.

Teaching individuals who have severe disabilities to use socially acceptable means of communicating what they want or do not want can take any number of forms. Depending on an individual's cognitive and motor skills as well as existing communication skills, the teaching may involve speech, manual signing, assistive devices, or idiosyncratic gestures. The primary concern is to teach individuals how to use the selected communication skill, as well as to teach individuals the appropriate conditions in which to use the communicative skill once learned.

In regard to using socially acceptable communication skills to get something that is desired, the focus may be on how to appropriately seek and maintain attention. When an individual uses challenging behavior such as aggression or disruption to gain attention, more appropriate communication skills such as greeting or requesting behaviors can replace the aggression or disruption for obtaining desired attention. In this manner, the individual is being taught functional *replacement behaviors*. Teaching and generally promoting replacement behaviors often comprise part of behavior support plans (see next chapter). Relatedly, the focus may be on teaching an individual to use acceptable communication skills to request or obtain a desired item instead of stealing, grabbing, or otherwise attempting to obtain the item with problem behavior.

Teaching functional communication skills to assist an individual to get out of something that is unwanted usually involves one or both of the following situations. The first situation is to allow an individual to avoid doing something that the individual does not want to do, without relying on challenging behavior to avoid the event. For example, instead of aggressing toward a staff member who requests or instructs an individual to do something undesired, the person might be taught to sign or gesture “no” or “not now”. The second situation is to allow the individual to get out of, or escape, an ongoing activity that becomes unpleasant for the individual without relying on problem behavior. In the latter situation, an individual might be taught to activate an adaptive device to indicate a desire for a break or to change to another activity. The latter communication skills could be used functionally to replace problem behavior that allows one to escape an activity by throwing materials involved in the ongoing activity, beginning to injure oneself, or aggressing toward a staff person.

As just indicated, teaching individuals functional communication skills to replace challenging behavior represents a critical component of many behavior support plans. However, the teaching process usually only represents a part of an overall plan. In some cases, it may not be appropriate to include teaching of replacement behavior in certain support plans. For example, teaching an appropriate way to communicate a desire to avoid or escape a given activity that is often accompanied by problem behavior may not be appropriate because the activity is something that is unavoidable. In such cases it is usually the responsibility of the author of the behavior support plan to determine other ways to overcome the problem behavior, such as by making the necessary activity more desirable. Nonetheless, teaching acceptable communication skills is typically an important option to consider when designing a support plan to overcome an existing problem behavior. Equally importantly, in almost every case, teaching functional communication skills can be a very useful preventive measure for reducing the likelihood that challenging behavior will develop in the first place.

Functional Skills to Teach to People Who Have Severe Disabilities Include:

1) **Skills involving activities that someone else would have to do for an individual if the individual could not do the activities**
2) **Skills that are needed and can be used frequently**
3) **Skills for which a person can be paid to perform as part of a job**
4) **Skills that allow a person to get something wanted or get out of something unwanted without problem behavior**

Special Considerations for Authors of Behavior Support Plans

Do Formal Programs Exist for Teaching Functional Skills?

There are many ways to teach functional skills to people with severe disabilities. One of the most common ways in congregate settings is by incorporating formal teaching programs that focus on functional skills within a consumer's individualized treatment plan (e.g., Individual Education Plan, Person-Centered Plan, Individual Program Plan). Each consumer treatment plan usually should include the teaching of functional skills as respective treatment goals.

Clinicians who are responsible for developing a support plan for a consumer's challenging behavior should ensure that formal programs for teaching skills that meet the functional guidelines described in this chapter exist in the consumer's comprehensive treatment plan. If, upon review of the consumer's individualized plan, a clinician finds that there are no identifiable goals for teaching functional skills, the clinician should advocate for the development of such goals and corresponding teaching programs.

It should also be noted though that the existence of formal teaching programs for functional skill development does not guarantee that respective consumers will actually be taught functional skills. The programs must be implemented consistently and effectively. However, when such programs do exist as part of overall treatment plans, they at least set the stage for functional teaching to occur.

Formal teaching programs also are advantageous in that they typically require collection of data to evaluate the progress of consumers in acquiring the target skills. Clinicians should review what programs exist, and how well a given individual is progressing on the programs as part of the process of developing behavior support plans for the consumer's challenging behavior. If such a review indicates that sufficient progress on the teaching programs is not occurring, then clinicians should advocate for a review of the teaching process to determine how the approach can be revised to be more effective. In many cases, lack of progress on teaching programs is due simply to the programs not being carried out as often as they are intended or need to be carried out.

It should be stressed to respective team members and appropriate agency executives that if there are not effective programs ongoing for teaching functional skills to consumers, then the overall environment is lacking a critical therapeutic component. It should likewise be stressed that without concerted attention to helping consumers develop functional skills, the occurrence of challenging behavior is likely to be a continuous concern, even if behavior support plans are developed.

The most common reason that people with severe disabilities do not learn the skills targeted in teaching programs is that the programs are not taught frequently enough

Do Consumers Routinely Participate in Functional Activities?

The importance of frequent participation in purposeful or functional activities on the overall welfare of individuals with severe disabilities, as well as on the prevention and treatment of challenging behavior, was stressed in **Chapter 4**. It was likewise noted that clinicians charged with developing support plans for a consumer's challenging behavior should review the degree to which the consumer regularly participates in functional activities. Such a review should take place *before* an individualized support plan is developed for the problem behavior. If the review indicates that a consumer has little involvement in functional activities, then changes in the consumer's routine and environment should be made in order to increase functional activity involvement.

A consumer's environment, including the teaching of functional skills, should be addressed before developing a support plan for a consumer's problem behavior because the behavior may be a direct result of a nontherapeutic environment. If a support plan is designed without correcting problems in the environment, then the basis for the problem behavior will not be sufficiently addressed and the plan is usually doomed to failure. As stressed previously, problem behavior cannot be treated in a problematic environment. If a consumer spends little time involved in purposeful activities and is not learning functional skills, then the environment represents a problem that needs correcting.

Where Do Consumers Participate in Day Treatment Activities?

A variable that often affects the types of activities in which consumers participate, as well as their degree of participation, is where day treatment activities are provided. Results of some research and a vast amount of experience indicate that individuals with severe disabilities are more likely to participate in functional activities if they attend such activities in environments that are geographically separate from their residences. Just as it is normal for adults without disabilities to work and participate in events outside of their homes on typical weekdays, it is usually more desirable for individuals with severe disabilities who live in congregate settings to attend work and other day programs outside of their residences.

For a variety of reasons, some human service agencies attempt to provide day treatment services for their consumers in the consumers' residences. For example, in a number of larger congregate living arrangements, it is viewed as more resource efficient to provide day treatment services within residences. The rationale is that it requires less personnel and related resources (e.g., transportation) to provide day services in the same place where consumers live. It is further reasoned that essentially, the same teaching, vocational, and other treatment services that would be provided in a workshop or adult activity center can be provided in the home. In other cases, it is not really a matter of resources but one of lack of effort; it is simply easier for staff not to have to work through transition duties of getting consumers transported out of the home for day services. In still other cases, and particularly in smaller community settings, consumers do not leave their group homes for day services because their agency has not found available day programs for them to attend in the local community.

Regardless of the reason for consumers remaining in their homes for day treatment services, the result is usually the same: there is less involvement in functional teaching activities relative to day programs provided outside of the home. When consumers go to sites outside of their residences for day services, by definition they have opportunities to experience a wider variety of settings during their weekdays. They also generally have increased opportunities to interact with more people both with and without disabilities, to learn new skills, and to be reinforced for using a wider variety of skills. In short, consumers are more likely to experience a meaningful day if their day-to-day existence is not restricted to one location. Meaningful days help promote meaningful behavior—behavior that is incompatible with problem behavior.

When consumer weekday activities are limited to the home environment, it is difficult to provide meaningful daily experiences and generally more likely that challenging behavior will occur

There are additional reasons why day treatment services provided within the residences of people with severe disabilities usually are less successful in teaching functional skills to consumers than day programs outside of the residences. One major reason is the impact of the location on the expectations and performance of support staff. Formal day treatment settings such as workshops and adult activity centers exist essentially exclusively to provide day treatment services. Staff are hired and usually supervised with the understanding that their role is to support consumers in participating in the activities provided. In contrast, in home environments, there are many other expectations of staff, ranging from providing personal care to arranging and supervising desired leisure activities.

Because of the wider variety of performance expectations of support staff in living settings, it is often more difficult to effectively establish and maintain functional teaching services in homes during the regular weekday. There seems to be a natural tendency for staff to spend more time on less teaching-oriented, passive pursuits in home environments relative to formal day programs. Such a tendency is evident when the home staff accompany consumers to a day program site to assist with treatment services in the latter setting. There is frequently a marked difference in staff performance in the two environments due to different performance expectations, intensity and focus of supervision, and availability of materials and resources to support vocational and other functional activities. Support staff usually spend more time teaching consumers and promoting purposeful activity involvement in the day program than the home environment.

In short, when considering the need for a behavior support plan for a respective consumer's challenging behavior, it is wise for the responsible clinician to review the degree to which the consumer has opportunities to participate in day treatment services in locations separate from the consumer's residence. If the consumer does not have a meaningful day treatment program in another location, it is also wise for the clinician to advocate for finding an off-site program that can be provided on a consistent basis.

How and When Teaching of Functional Skills Occurs

Earlier it was noted that the existence of formal teaching programs as part of a consumer's individualized program plan is an important but not sufficient requirement for successful teaching of functional skills. The programs must be effectively implemented. It was likewise noted that a common reason that teaching programs do not result in consumers learning the skills targeted in the programs is that the teaching does not occur frequently enough. Hence, clinicians, supervisors, and other agency personnel responsible for developing and overseeing behavior support plans for challenging behavior should review both the existence of formal teaching programs and the effectiveness of the programs. If programs are not resulting in consumer acquisition of functional skills, then the frequency with which the programs are implemented should be reviewed.

When conducting a review of teaching services, it is likewise important to consider *how* the programs are carried out. Of course, the programs should be designed with sound teaching strategies and the programs should be carried out in the manner they are written. However, there are also two more general ways to consider in regard to how teaching programs are implemented. One way is during formal, circumscribed teaching sessions in which a staff person schedules time to work with a respective consumer to conduct the consumer's program. A second way is to incorporate teaching of the targeted skills within the consumer's daily routine whenever the consumer could naturally use the skill. The latter teaching format represents a *naturalistic* approach to teaching functional skills. To be most effective for assisting consumers in learning functional skills and reducing the occurrence of challenging behavior, teaching programs usually should be carried out in both ways.

Implementing teaching programs in both a formal and naturalistic format is particularly important in regard to teaching replacement skills. To review briefly, replacement skills refer to socially appropriate skills that are taught to consumers to replace the need for the consumers to use problem behavior to meet their needs. In many settings, several concerns typically warrant the attention of clinicians and other personnel responsible for behavior support plans regarding how replacement skills are taught. One concern is when a specified replacement skill is designed to be taught only when a consumer engages in the problem behavior that is desired to be replaced. This situation occurs when the replacement skill is identified in a behavior support plan with instructions for staff to, for example, prompt and reinforce the occurrence of the replacement behavior when the consumer begins to display the problem behavior. To illustrate, a support plan may indicate that when a consumer begins to aggress during an ongoing activity, the staff person should prompt the consumer to say or sign "break".

Attempting to teach a replacement skill to a consumer in the type of situation just illustrated can be useful. However, it should not be the only time that teaching occurs with the individual. People with severe disabilities often need considerable practice and opportunities to be reinforced for learning and using a particular skill. If the skill is only taught when the consumer engages in a problem behavior, the teaching is likely to be too infrequent to have much success. Additionally, in many cases once the problem behavior is initiated, the consumer already achieves at least part of the desired outcome such that there is little reason for the consumer to use the alternative replacement skill. In other cases it simply is too difficult to interrupt the problem behavior once it begins in order to teach a more appropriate behavior.

Another concern that occurs in regard to teaching specific replacement skills for challenging behavior is that although the teaching process is written into a consumer's overall treatment plan and teaching is scheduled to take place, very little teaching actually occurs. The primary reason that scheduled teaching of replacement behaviors does not occur is that support staff and other agency personnel are not sufficiently aware of the importance of the teaching. Staff are usually quite aware of a given consumer's problem behavior, and know the importance of responding to the behavior in a certain way as prescribed in the consumer's support plan. Challenging behavior is usually quite apparent to staff, and the need to eliminate the behavior is also quite apparent. However, the fact that the consumer is not displaying appropriate skills to meet the needs being met by the problem behavior is not so apparent to staff. Correspondingly, the importance of teaching appropriate replacement skills is not very apparent. In essence, challenging behavior typically draws staff attention and action much more readily than the lack of appropriate behavior. This represents a major reason that teaching of functional skills is often overlooked in the overall process of preventing and treating challenging behavior.

To overcome lack of attention directed to teaching replacement skills, clinicians responsible for behavior support plans must make concerted efforts to impress upon staff the importance of spending time teaching consumers specific replacement skills. It is likewise important that staffs' performance in teaching replacement skills be closely supervised. Methods of providing supervision are provided in subsequent chapters. The point here is that clinicians should be aware that the teaching of replacement skills as part of an overall plan to overcome challenging behavior frequently is not given the attention necessary to ensure that the teaching occurs in an effective manner.

Clinicians should be especially vigilant about the teaching of replacement skills as part of a support plan for challenging behavior; this component of a plan is often carried out less consistently than other parts of the plan

Another reason that teaching replacement behaviors is often neglected relative to other parts of treatment plans is due to how responsibility of implementing aspects of the plans is divided among a consumer's support team members. In many agencies, certain clinical staff such as psychologists are responsible for reducing challenging behavior. Other clinicians such as teachers are responsible for teaching adaptive skills. Hence, when it is determined that a specific replacement skill should be taught as one component of a behavior support plan, that responsibility is assigned to someone other than the clinician who developed the plan. For example, if the replacement behavior is a communicative skill, such as requesting to stop an ongoing activity, the responsibility to develop and implement a teaching strategy may be assigned to a speech/language pathologist.

In the example just illustrated, often the clinician who is assigned the responsibility of teaching the replacement skill does not place a very high priority on the responsibility relative to other duties. The lower priority occurs because the clinician is more concerned about teaching skills that are based on his or her clinical view of what needs to be done, and not what is dictated by another clinician (in this case, the clinician who developed the support plan for the problem behavior that includes teaching of a replacement skill). The end result is that little attention is directed to ensuring that a necessary replacement skill is effectively taught.

There are other reasons that teaching of replacement skills receives less attention relative to other components of behavior support plans. However, the two reasons just summarized generally are the most common. In any case, clinicians as well as staff supervisors need to be aware that this aspect of preventing and treating challenging behavior usually requires close scrutiny and supervision.

SECTION III

SETTING THE OCCASION FOR EFFECTIVE IMPLEMENTATION OF BEHAVIOR SUPPORT PLANS: ESSENTIAL PROGRAM COMPONENTS AND STAFF TRAINING PROCEDURES

CHAPTER 6

Essential Components of Behavior Support Plans for Overcoming Challenging Behavior

In the introductory comments to this manual it was noted that a critical element in the prevention and treatment of challenging behavior is the availability of a quality support plan. Even when environments in which individuals with severe disabilities live, work, and play have all the desirable attributes as discussed in the preceding chapters, some individuals may still display challenging behavior. When challenging behavior does occur, a sound support plan is necessary to help overcome the problem behavior.

As also discussed previously, tremendous progress has occurred in the last two decades in developing a technology for treating challenging behavior among people with severe disabilities. That technology includes a wide array of behavior change procedures that can be incorporated within treatment plans. On a general level though, the numerous procedures can be grouped into a few key categories based on whether they are used prior to the occurrence of problem behavior versus after the behavior occurs. Procedures used in the former situation are intended to prevent the problem behavior from occurring. Procedures used in the latter situation are intended to reduce the likelihood that the problem behavior will be repeated.

This chapter summarizes the key categories of behavior change procedures that constitute treatment or support plans for challenging behavior among people with severe disabilities. The intent is to provide basic information regarding what to expect in a support plan if that plan is to include currently recommended practices regarding the prevention and treatment of challenging behavior. In particular, the intent is to describe what someone should ask of a treatment plan, and the procedural information that should be obtainable from the plan to allow staff to adequately carry out the treatment procedures.

Before discussing the key components of effective support plans for challenging behavior, it should be noted that the purpose of this chapter is not to describe how to actually develop treatment plans. Such a task would require a text in and of itself. For readers interested in more detailed information on developing support plans for challenging behavior among people with severe disabilities, the **Selected Readings** provide a number of highly regarded books and manuals (see section on **Developing Quality Behavior Support Plans**). Again, the intent here is to describe what to expect of behavior support plans, and what information should be obtainable from respective plans to allow staff to implement the plans effectively.

Assessing Likely Reasons Why Challenging Behavior Occurs

One of the most notable advances in preventing and treating challenging behavior has been the recent development of procedures for determining variables that occasion problem behavior. A variety of *functional assessment* procedures have been developed for determining the function that challenging behavior serves for an individual—that is, an individual's reason or motivation for the behavior. As discussed in previous chapters, a very large amount of challenging behavior among individuals with severe disabilities functions as a means to: (1) obtain something an individual wants such as attention from others or a desired item or, (2) avoid something that an individual does not want such as to participate in an ongoing activity or respond to a directive from a support person. The determination that challenging behavior usually occurs for at least one of these reasons is a direct result of research and application with functional assessment procedures.

Prior to the advent of functional assessment methodologies, treatment plans for challenging behavior did not always address an individual's reason for engaging in the behavior. The plans simply focused on changing the behavior, or reducing its frequency. There is now a professional consensus that behavior support plans are more likely to have long-term success if the plans are developed in consideration of an individual's motivation for displaying the problem behavior.

People with severe disabilities usually display problem behavior because the behavior serves the purpose or function of getting something the individuals want, or avoiding something the individuals do not want

Currently, recommended practice generally requires that some type of functional assessment be completed prior to developing a treatment plan for challenging behavior. The purpose here though is not to describe how to conduct functional assessments as part of the development of behavior support plans; that responsibility usually rests with a psychologist or other clinician who writes the plan (information pertaining to functional assessment methodologies is provided in references in the **Selected Readings** on **Developing Quality Behavior Support Plans**). From the perspective of knowing what to expect to be in treatment plans however, as well as to be able to obtain necessary information from the plans to allow direct service staff to adequately implement the plans, two key issues related to functional assessments warrant attention. The first issue relates to the involvement of direct support staff in the functional assessment process. The second issue pertains to ensuring that behavior change procedures encompassed within a treatment plan relate to an individual's motivation for engaging in the behavior of concern.

Involving Staff in the Determination of an Individual's Motivation for Problem Behavior

As just indicated, there are a number of functional assessment procedures for identifying an individual's motivation for engaging in challenging behavior. It is usually the responsibility of the person who develops the support plan to determine which type of functional assessment is most relevant in a respective situation. To enhance the proficiency with which direct service staff eventually implement the treatment plan that is developed, it is important that the staff be involved in whatever functional assessment process is used.

There are a variety of ways direct support staff can be involved in functional assessment processes used to identify why an individual displays challenging behavior. Most importantly though, direct support personnel should have opportunities to express their opinion as to why an individual engages in problem behavior. Direct service staff should always be questioned by clinicians who develop behavior support plans regarding what they think motivates the individual to act in a certain way.

There are two primary reasons why the opinions of support staff should be solicited in regard to why a consumer displays problem behavior. First, because these staff generally spend the most time with consumers who have severe disabilities in congregate settings, they usually know the consumers better than anyone else in the service agency. As a result, direct support staff are in an opportune position to provide valuable insight regarding what motivates an individual to display challenging behavior. These staff can also provide detailed information about the situations in which an individual is most and least likely to display the problem behavior—information that can be critical for conducting a successful functional assessment.

A second reason why direct support personnel should be involved in the functional assessment process is perhaps less apparent than obtaining relevant information for developing a treatment plan, but is no less important. By involving staff in the process and soliciting as well as attending to their opinions, staff willingness to carry out a plan once developed can be enhanced. Staff are often more willing to carry out various work duties if they have an active role in determining and structuring those duties. In the case of conducting functional assessments for developing a behavior support plan, staff involvement in the process helps ensure staff are aware of the rationale for the plan and are in agreement with the specific procedures to be applied.

Skilled clinicians who develop behavior support plans always incorporate the views of direct service staff in the functional assessment process as well as in the subsequent development of the plans. Other clinicians tend to develop treatment plans with little or no regard for staff views. Whether due to time constraints, oversight based on inexperience, or feelings of professional territoriality (i.e., the view that only a trained professional such as a licensed psychologist should be involved in developing treatment plans), the latter process invariably decreases the likelihood that staff will be receptive to carrying out a support plan.

When staff do not have opportunities to express their opinions regarding why an individual engages in problem behavior, or their opinions are not attended to in the development of a support plan, they are much more likely to express concerns over the viability or likely effectiveness of the plan. These concerns can detract from staffs' motivation to implement the plan consistently and effectively. Such concerns can also result in overt disgruntlement with the plan as well as with the clinician who developed the plan. Staff discontent regarding a support plan and the responsible clinician almost always causes serious problems with implementation of the plan and subsequently, the plan's effectiveness. This type of situation can likewise make the clinician's future work related to treatment of problem behavior much more difficult.

Opinions of direct service staff should always be attended to when assessing an individual's motivation for problem behavior, and when developing a support plan

Essential Components of Behavior Support Plans

From the perspective of staff implementation of behavior support plans, there are four components or categories of procedures that usually should be included in the plans. The first component involves clear specification of the consumer's *behavior* that the plan is intended to decrease, as well as the behavior that is intended to be increased. The second component is *environmental set-ups*, or those procedures that should and should not be in place in the routine environments of people with severe disabilities in order to reduce the likelihood that problem behavior will occur. The third component pertains to *antecedents*, which are events that often occur immediately before an individual engages in a given problem behavior. With this component, what staff should do if the antecedents occur should be specified in the plan. Finally, the fourth component involves responses or *consequences* that staff should provide when the behaviors to decrease and the behaviors to increase are observed.

Essential Components of Behavior Support Plans I: Specification of Behaviors to Decrease and Increase

The development of support plans for challenging behavior essentially begins with identification of target behaviors. Target behaviors represent what the plans are intended to change. More specifically, the plans are intended to alter how frequently the behaviors occur, or in which situations the behaviors occur. Clearly specifying a consumer's target behaviors to change represents the first essential component that should be included in a behavior support plan.

The importance of clearly articulating what behaviors are intended to be changed by a support plan is generally well accepted among psychologists and other clinicians who develop treatment plans for challenging behavior. On occasion though, direct support staff are presented with a treatment plan that does not adequately specify the behaviors to change. Lack of appropriate specification frequently occurs with problem behavior that is of a social nature. For example, a plan might refer to reducing a consumer's socially offensive language. Socially offensive language can mean different things to different people, depending in part on personal value systems among staff, cultural differences, or individual learning histories among staff. If staff have differing views regarding what constitutes socially offensive language, then they are likely to implement a given support plan differently. When various staff implement a plan differently with a consumer, then the plan is almost always doomed to failure.

To help ensure that direct support staff implement a treatment plan consistently, it is incumbent upon the author of the plan to clearly specify the target behaviors to decrease. Staff as well as their supervisors should be able to look at a plan and readily answer the question, "*What are the target behaviors to decrease or to have occur less often*?". One straightforward means of checking to make sure the target behaviors to decrease are appropriately specified is to ask this question of staff who have reviewed the plan. If staff answer the question in the same way, then the behaviors have probably been sufficiently specified. In contrast, if staff identify different behaviors in response to the question, or have difficulty naming any consumer behaviors to decrease, then the plan probably needs to be revised to better specify the behaviors that are intended to be decreased.

Although target behaviors to be decreased are usually well specified in current treatment plans for challenging behavior with some exceptions as just illustrated, there are other target behaviors that tend to be less well specified. The latter behaviors pertain to what the plans are intended to increase on the part of a consumer. In most situations, the target behaviors to be increased in frequency by a support plan are just as important as the behaviors to be decreased.

As indicated previously, a professional consensus exists that a functional assessment should be completed as part of the development of a behavior support plan. One intent of a functional assessment is to identify more appropriate means for an individual to achieve a desired function or purpose that is currently being achieved through problem behavior. Often the latter intent is to teach or otherwise support an individual in using socially acceptable behavior to achieve the desired function. The socially acceptable behavior, or *replacement behavior* (see **Chapter 5**) that the individual can use to replace the problem behavior usually represents the behavior that should be increased in frequency as part of a treatment plan.

If direct service staff are to be expected to implement a behavior support plan in an appropriate and effective manner, then the consumer behaviors to be increased must be clearly specified. Staff must be able to look at a respective support plan and readily answer the same type of question as that noted earlier, only this time the question pertains to "*What are the behaviors to increase*?". Unless all staff who are charged with implementing a treatment plan can answer the question correctly, the plan is not likely to be implemented effectively and needs to be revised.

Quality behavior support plans clearly specify a consumer's behavior to decrease *and* a consumer's behavior to increase

Essential Components of Behavior Support Plans II: Environmental Set-Ups

Environmental set-ups are referred to in different ways in treatment plans for challenging behavior. Some plans refer to this component as preventive procedures or setting events. However, we prefer to call this component environmental set-ups because it pertains to what should and should not be in place in an individual's environment—or how the environment should be *set up* to prevent or at least reduce the likelihood that the problem behavior will occur. Because what should be in place as well as what should not be in place are both important aspects of environmental set-ups, the following sections discuss each respective aspect.

Environmental Set-Ups Regarding What Should Be in Place

Each behavior support plan should identify specific features of the environment of an individual that make it unlikely that the individual's problem behavior will occur. For many people with severe disabilities, this type of environmental set-up involves having ready access to preferred leisure items during typical leisure or recreational times. Access to preferred leisure items can be an important environmental set-up because the presence of the items, or the individual's interactions with the items, is often associated with an absence of problem behavior. For other individuals, and particularly people whose problem behavior serves the purpose of gaining attention from others, environmental set-ups to have in place involve frequent social exchanges with other people such as direct support staff. For these individuals, frequent social interactions can be associated with desirable behavior by the individuals and an absence or reduced occurrence of problem behavior.

There are many other types of environmental set-ups that can be included in behavior support plans. The specific items, events, or activities that are desired to be in place in the environment of a given individual can usually be derived from various types of functional assessments. Regardless of what constitutes the appropriate environmental set-ups that should be routinely present though, the set-ups should be specifically identified in the plans. Sometimes plans need to specify different environmental set-ups that need to be in place in different locations that an individual frequents on a daily basis, such as in the individual's group home versus where the individual works.

In some cases, support plans refer to environmental set-ups in one format or another, but lack sufficient specification to ensure that staff and supervisors know exactly what should be present. To ensure support plans adequately specify environmental set-ups to be present, supervisors and staff should be able to read the plans and answer the question "*What things should be in place in the everyday environment of the individual to reduce the likelihood of problem behavior*?". The environmental set-ups should also be specified to the degree that a supervisor (or author of the behavior support plan) can walk into an individual's environment and immediately determine whether the things that should be in place are indeed present. If a supervisor cannot answer this question, or cannot make a quick observational determination regarding the environmental set-ups, then the behavior support plan probably needs to be revised to include more specificity.

Environmental Set-Ups Regarding What Should Not Be in Place

In addition to identifying what should be in place to reduce the probability that challenging behavior will occur, behavior support plans should identify what should not be in place. For example, for some individuals with severe disabilities, crowded or loud environments are often accompanied by certain problem behaviors. For those individuals, their support plans need to specify that they should be assisted in avoiding crowded or loud situations; that is, large crowds or unusually loud noises should not be present in their routine environments. For other persons, certain types of instructions or directives by staff are accompanied by problem behavior. For those persons, support plans should indicate that these types of instructions and directives should not be provided by staff (or the plans should identify other means of providing the instructions and directives that are less likely to occasion problem behavior).

As with environmental set-ups that should be in place, those things that should not be routinely present in an individual's environment must be well specified in a behavior support plan. Supervisors and staff should be able to read the plan and readily answer the question, "*What should not be present in this consumer's day-to-day environment*?". Additionally, these types of environmental set-ups should be specified in the plan to the degree that a supervisor or clinician can walk into a consumer's environment and quickly determine if things that should not be present are indeed absent from the environment.

Environmental set-ups should be specified in support plans such that supervisors and clinicians can enter a consumer's routine environment and quickly determine if things that should be present are indeed present *and* things that should not be in the environment are not present

Essential Components of Behavior Support Plans III: Antecedents

A third essential component of behavior support plans involves antecedents to target behaviors. Antecedents refer to events that tend to happen right before an individual engages in a particular behavior. Put another way, when an antecedent event for a certain behavior occurs, then it is likely that the behavior will be displayed. When considering problem behavior, antecedents generally refer to events that occur right before a problem behavior, and make it more likely that the problem behavior will occur (i.e., relative to the situation in which the antecedent event does not happen).

Any number of events can represent antecedents for problem behavior among people who have severe disabilities. For some individuals, a change in the usual or predicted daily routine, such as a work placement being canceled for the day, can be an antecedent for problem behavior. For other individuals, a request or instruction from a support staff to do an undesired activity can be an antecedent event for subsequent problem behavior.

Antecedents to problem behavior should be clearly identified in behavior support plans whenever possible. Knowledge about antecedents to problem behavior can help prevent the behavior from occurring. Such knowledge can help prevent problem behavior in two ways. First, support staff can prevent the antecedent event from taking place. For example, if an antecedent for a consumer's aggressive behavior is observing another consumer receive explicit praise from a staff person (which could set the occasion for the former consumer to become aggressive in an attempt to gain attention from the staff person), one way to prevent the antecedent from occurring might be to provide praise to the other consumer in a private manner that is out of view of other people.

A second way that awareness of antecedents can prevent problem behavior pertains not to preventing the antecedent from occurring, but to changing what the consumer is doing when the event happens. In a number of cases, support staff will not be able to prevent antecedent events from happening. To illustrate, an antecedent event for a consumer's self-injurious face slapping might be when another individual sits too close to the consumer on a sofa or other seating arrangement. In this case, staff may not be able, or may not want, to prevent the individual from sitting there. However, staff may still be able to prevent the self-injury from occurring by immediately interacting with the consumer and involving the consumer in another activity, perhaps in another area of the room. By involving the consumer in another activity and redirecting the consumer's attention away from the individual who just sat down, it becomes less likely that the consumer will display the problem behavior.

Awareness of antecedents to problem behavior can help prevent the behavior from occurring by allowing staff to make it less likely that an antecedent event happens, and by allowing staff to change what the consumer is doing if the antecedent does occur

In order for direct support staff to make use of knowledge of antecedent events to help prevent challenging behavior from occurring, what constitutes the antecedents must be well specified in treatment plans. A staff person should be able to look at the plan and readily answer the question, "*What often occurs right before a problem behavior for this consumer?*". Equally importantly, and particularly from the perspective of implementing the treatment plan, one should be able to look at the plan and immediately answer the question, "*When the antecedent event for a certain problem behavior occurs, what should be done to prevent the behavior from happening?*". If either of these questions cannot be answered by reviewing the behavior support plan, then the author of the plan should be consulted and the plan revised whenever possible.

In considering information about antecedents to problem behavior as a necessary component of behavior support plans, a practical qualification warrants mentioning. In some situations, there is no apparent antecedent to a problem behavior, or at least the antecedent has not been identified. When authors of behavior support plans, in conjunction with input from direct service staff, are unable to identify antecedents to problem behavior, then this component cannot be included within a support plan. In this situation, the plan should specify that antecedents to the behavior have not been identified.

Essential Components of Behavior Support Plans IV: What to Do When the Behaviors to Decrease and Increase Occur

The final component that is an essential part of quality support plans for challenging behavior involves specification of what staff should do when a consumer's target behaviors are observed. Because target behaviors refer both to what is desired for the consumer to do less often as well as more often, how staff should respond to both types of behavior must be specified in the plan. The intent is for staff to be able to respond in a way that reinforces the behaviors identified to be increased, and to avoid reinforcing the behaviors to be decreased.

Similar to specification of target behaviors to be decreased and increased as discussed earlier, support plans usually include better specification about what staff should do in response to a behavior to decrease than a behavior to increase. Typically plans sufficiently specify that when a consumer displays a certain problem behavior that is intended to be decreased, staff should do something such as interrupt the behavior, withdraw their attention, redirect the consumer to another activity, engage the consumer in relaxation activities, etc. Nevertheless, it is still helpful to make sure support plans clearly specify staff action in response to observed consumer behaviors to decrease. Staff should be able to review the plan and readily answer the question, "*When the consumer displays* (a target behavior to decrease), *what should be done*?".

In contrast to specification of what staff should do when a consumer's behavior to decrease occurs, specification of staff actions in response to behaviors to increase is provided inconsistently in many behavior support plans. To illustrate, in a support plan designed to help an individual overcome aggressive behavior that serves the function of allowing the individual to discontinue a certain activity, the plan may indicate that staff should respond to the consumer's desire to take a break or stop the activity prior to any aggression. In this case, an appropriate means of requesting a break may represent the behavior to increase, in contrast to the consumer hitting the staff member as a means of getting out of the activity (the latter behavior would of course represent the behavior to decrease). However, such a plan fails to specify the behaviors that a consumer can use to indicate a desired break, as well as what staff should do to provide a break for the consumer. Some staff may interpret the plan to mean that the consumer must say or sign something like "I want to stop" or simply "stop". Other staff may interpret the plan to mean that any indication the consumer is becoming tired of the activity is sufficient, such as the consumer yawning, beginning to attend to other things in the room rather than the activity, or simply taking longer to complete aspects of the activity. Relatedly, some staff may provide a break by terminating the activity whereas other staff may provide a break by temporarily discontinuing the activity for only a minute or two.

In the situation just illustrated, different staff would likely respond to different behaviors by the consumer, and respond in contrasting ways to a given behavior. Different staff would provide various types of breaks based on different things the consumer did (e.g., sign "break" versus yawn). Such inconsistency on the part of staff can make it difficult for a consumer to learn an appropriate way to express discontent with an activity, which makes it more likely the consumer will revert to using aggressive behavior to get out of the activity. The end result is that the behavior support plan is implemented inconsistently, and the plan is not likely to be effective.

To avoid inconsistency in implementing aspects of support plans designed to increase desired target behaviors, staff should be able to look at a plan and quickly determine what they should do if the consumer displays the behavior to be increased. All staff should be able to answer the question, "*What should be done if the consumer does* (<u>the behavior to increase</u>)?". Unless all staff who are responsible for implementing the behavior support plan can answer the question in the correct manner, it is unlikely the plan will be implemented effectively.

Preparing Behavior Support Plans to Facilitate Staff Implementation

Preceding sections summarized the key components that should comprise a support plan for challenging behavior among individuals with severe disabilities. There are other ways to summarize or categorize important components of behavior support plans. However, this particular way is usually advantageous for facilitating staff implementation of the plans. If staff and supervisors can answer the questions raised in the preceding sections regarding each key component of a behavior support plan, then the plan is probably appropriately thorough and staff will have a good understanding about how to implement the plan. A summary of the questions that support staff should be able to answer in order to adequately carry out behavior support plans is illustrated in the following **Behavior Support Plan Summary Form**.

The **Summary Form** can be a useful instrument to give to staff to help them obtain necessary procedural information from behavior support plans. The form can also be a useful aid when initially training staff to implement a given support plan (see **Chapter 7**) and when monitoring staffs' implementation of the plan (**Chapters 8** and **9**). The form can help staff and supervisors alike focus on those parts of behavior support plans that relate directly to what staff should do to fulfill their implementation duties associated with the plans.

When considering using the **Behavior Support Plan Summary Form** or a similar means of assisting staff in obtaining procedural information from a support plan, a frequent problem that arises is the way plans are written. Many behavior support plans for people with severe disabilities are written in a way that makes it difficult for staff to readily obtain information that specifies what they should do to implement the plans. Special consideration is warranted among psychologists and other authors of treatment plans to ensure that relevant procedural information is clear and accessible for staff who are charged with carrying out the plans. The following sections provide several guidelines that can be helpful when writing support plans to ensure procedural information is readily accessible to staff.

Behavior Support Plan Summary Form

Consumer name:________________ Date plan begins:__________

Target Behaviors

What are the behaviors to decrease?

What are the behaviors to increase?

Environmental Set-ups

What should be present in the everyday environment?

What should not be present in the everyday environment?

Antecedents

What event often happens right before a problem behavior?

What should be done if the event happens?

Consequences

What should be done if the behavior to decrease occurs?

What should be done if the behavior to increase occurs?

Figure 6-1: *Behavior Support Plan Summary Form* for summarizing staff implementation information from a behavior support plan for an individual's challenging behavior. Drawn from Reid, D.H., Parsons, M.B., Rotholz, D.A., Braswell, B.A., & Morris, L.A. (in press). *The Carolina Curriculum on Positive Behavior Support: Supervisory Edition*. Washington, D.C.: American Association on Mental Retardation.

Ensuring Information On Implementation Procedures is Readily Accessible Within Behavior Support Plans

Behavior support plans for people with severe disabilities and challenging behavior often include a considerable amount of written information. It is common, for example, to find behavior support plans that range from 5 to 25 typed pages in length. Much of the information included in the plans does not pertain to what staff should do to carry out the plans. Plans frequently include such information as a description of the consumer, the consumer's background history, existing living arrangement, current medication regime, and a summary of previous assessments and treatment plans. This type of information is useful in various ways, but its presence in a support plan makes it difficult for staff to find the specifics of what they are expected to do to implement the plan.

Generally it is most useful if staff can pick up a behavior support plan and immediately read exactly what they need to do to carry out the plan. Direct service staff in congregate settings for people who have severe disabilities often are responsible for groups of consumers, and are expected to implement behavior support plans for a number of consumers. These staff also are expected to carry out treatment plans developed in areas other than those related to challenging behavior, such as plans developed by education personnel for teaching adaptive skills, speech and language pathologists for enhancing communication skills, and physical or occupational therapists for promoting motor development. Hence, direct service staff must be familiar with a number of different types of treatment plans. If the plans are not written in a way that makes it easy to find specifics about implementation, it is unlikely that staff will have the time (or in some cases, the motivation) to read and study every plan for every consumer to find relevant information for carrying out each plan.

In one sense, the problem of implementation information not being readily accessible in a behavior support plan would seem to be remedied in a straight forward fashion: simply limit the written plan to information that is necessary to implement the plan. On closer examination though, the solution is more complicated. People who write behavior support plans must respond to a number of expectations regarding the type of information provided in support plans. Professional standards typically require relevant background information about the consumer, previous assessment and treatment results, etc. Regulatory standards in educational agencies and certain types of residential settings also require various types of information to be present in behavior support plans beyond what is necessary to actually carry out the plans. In short, in many cases authors of behavior support plans are expected or required to write lengthy plans that include much more information than what is needed to implement the plans.

When considering expectations placed on authors of behavior support plans in terms of everything that must be included in the plans, as well as the need to make implementation information readily accessible to staff, treatment plan authors have a serious dilemma. The dilemma is whether to: (1) write a plan in a comprehensive and lengthy manner to coincide with professional and regulatory expectations, while knowing that such a format makes it difficult for direct service staff to read and understand the plan or, (2) write a plan in a succinct format focusing exclusively on what should be done to carry out the plan to facilitate staff implementation, while knowing that this format may not meet professional or regulatory standards.

There does not appear to be an ideal solution to the dilemma just noted. One recommended approach involves authors of behavior support plans preparing two versions of a support plan. One version, which represents the behavior support plan proper, includes all the information that is expected to be in the plan. The second version, which represents in essence a behavior support plan procedural summary, simply describes what must be done to carry out the plan. The former version usually goes into the consumer's official file or record, while the latter version is provided to staff. Staff can then review the lengthier version of the plan at their convenience if they so choose.

The process of preparing two versions of a behavior support plan can resolve the dilemma of what to include in a written plan. However, this approach is not ideal because it creates more work on the part of psychologists and other authors of behavior support plans. In essence, whoever develops a support plan must duplicate aspects of the development process in order to prepare two versions of the plan. Nevertheless, currently this approach appears to be the best option. The process can be expedited in many cases if a tool such as the **Behavior Support Plan Summary Form** described earlier is used as the implementation version of the plan. The **Summary Form** can be completed in a manner that includes all essential implementation information and then the form can be made readily available to staff.

Minimizing Technical Jargon When Writing Behavior Support Plans

Similar to the problem with too much information in a support plan making it difficult for staff to determine how to implement the plan, how the information is worded in the plan can impact staffs' understanding of procedural information. In particular, reliance on technical terminology or jargon can make staffs' task of reviewing and understanding the plan unnecessarily difficult. It must be remembered that most direct service staff have high school backgrounds, not college or university backgrounds. Even among the relatively few staff who have undergraduate experience, the experience is rarely in a field related to the backgrounds of clinicians who write behavior support plans. Technical terminology that is specific to a particular professional field such as behavioral psychology is not a part of other disciplines constituting undergraduate education. Terms such a negative reinforcement, stimulus control, and escape/avoidance that are commonly used among authors of behavior support plans are essentially foreign to everybody else. Consequently, any written version of a plan that is expected to be reviewed by staff should be void of this type of terminology.

Similar to the dilemma of deciding what type and how much information to put in plans, attempting to minimize technical terminology can put authors of support plans in a difficult position. Some information that is required in a plan is hard to provide without technical terms. The recommended solution to this apparent dilemma for people who write behavior support plans is similar to that just noted regarding the type and amount of information that go into a plan. Technical terminology should be limited to the version of the plan that is used for the consumer's file and regulatory purposes. The terminology should be avoided in the version that is given to staff.

Behavior support plans provided to direct service staff should be written in a way that facilitates staffs' obtainment of information on how to carry out the plans; the plans should be written succinctly and in every day language

CHAPTER 7

Essential Procedures for Training Staff to Implement Behavior Support Plans

Once a sound behavior support plan is developed, it is necessary to train staff how to implement the plan. As noted in previous chapters, the importance of training staff how to carry out behavior support plans is well accepted among most staff supervisors and clinicians who write the plans. However, the thoroughness and effectiveness with which training is conducted often leaves much to be desired. If training is to be truly effective such that everyone who is expected to implement the plan is well skilled in the necessary procedures, the training must be *competency-* and *performance-based.*

Competency-based staff training means that what staff are expected to learn in terms of target competencies is clearly specified prior to training, and training is not considered complete until staff demonstrate those competencies. Performance-based staff training is similar to competency-based training, but with more of an explicit focus on skill performance. That is, what staff are expected to do is carefully performed or demonstrated by whoever trains the staff and subsequently, by the staff trainees. Competency- and performance-based training can be conducted simultaneously, and a well-established means of conducting such training is available for human service personnel.

A Step-By-Step Process for Conducting Competency- and Performance-Based Staff Training

Competency- and performance-based staff training can be conducted in a very effective manner by following six basic steps. The steps comprising this approach to staff training are summarized below.

Component Steps of Competency- and Performance-Based Training

Step 1: Verbally describe the skills to be taught and a rationale for training the skills

Step 2: Provide a succinct, written description of the skills to be taught

Step 3: Demonstrate how to perform each skill

Step 4: Observe as trainees practice performing each skill

Step 5: Provide feedback to staff regarding their proficiency in performing each skill

Step 6: Repeat steps 3-5 until each staff trainee demonstrates proficiency in performing each skill

---

The six steps comprising effective staff training can be used to train essentially any performance skill expected of human service staff, including general practices involved in positive behavior support (e.g., preventive and therapeutic procedures to have in place in a given environment as discussed in **Chapters 3 - 5**) as well as carrying out individualized behavior support plans. A description of each training step is provided in the following chapter sections, along with how the steps relate specifically to training staff to carry out individualized behavior support plans.

Step 1: Describe the Skills to Be Taught

Training of performance skills to staff should begin with a rationale regarding why the target skills will be taught along with a precise description of what exactly the skills involve. A rationale is provided to give trainees a context within which to place the training, and to let them know why they will be expected to perform the skills that are being trained. Knowing the rationale and purpose behind the new expectations can enhance staff acceptance of the training as well as their potential motivation to perform the designated skills during their work routine. In contrast, if staff are simply told that they are to do something in the work place without an accompanying rationale, their subsequent motivation to perform the new duties can be diminished. In regard to being trained to implement a behavior support plan, if staff have been involved in the design of the plan as described in **Chapter 6**, typically the rationale is already apparent to staff. Hence, only a brief reference to the reason for the plan is necessary.

A precise verbal description of the target skills that will be trained is important to help ensure staff know exactly what is expected of them. The verbal description also supplements the written version of the target skills (**Step 2** of the training). Additionally, it is likely that in a number of settings, some staff may not read particularly well. In the latter situations, the verbal description of the target skills is especially important for staffs' understanding of their new performance expectations.

Step 2: Provide a Written Description of the Skills to Be Trained

Once the target skills of the training have been described for staff trainees, the next step in the training process is to provide a written summary of the skills. Providing a written summary of the new skills that staff are expected to perform as a result of training is advantageous in two ways. First, it reinforces what was explained verbally to staff in **Step 1**. Second, the summary represents a permanent product for staff to maintain and review as needed. In this way, staff who forget or are otherwise unsure what to do on the job after training can review the written summary to refresh their memory. Although some staff who forget what should be done in a particular circumstance will not be sufficiently motivated to review the form, other staff will be so motivated. For the latter staff, immediate availability of a written summary of their performance expectations can provide them with the desired information.

Generally, the best way to prepare a written summary of the skills being trained is to simply list only the specific things that staff must know how to do in order to fulfill their new performance responsibility. Providing information beyond what staff must specifically do tends to make the learning process more cumbersome, and can make it difficult for some staff to identify those specific duties that they must complete. One effective way to prepare a summary in this manner is to develop a *performance checklist* of the skills being trained. A checklist is in essence a task analysis of the exact steps staff must perform to carry out the skills targeted by the training, similar to the way a skill that is to be taught to an individual with a cognitive disability is task analyzed into its component behavioral steps. The steps comprising the staff training process as illustrated in the table presented previously in this chapter exemplifies one type of performance checklist—in this case, a checklist for staff trainers.

When training staff how to implement a respective consumer's behavior support plan, one means of preparing a concise written summary of the things that staff will need to do is by using the **Behavior Support Plan Summary Form** described in **Chapter 6**. To prepare the **Summary Form**, the staff trainer or author of the plan simply fills in the blanks regarding what staff should know and do in regard to behaviors to increase and decrease, environmental set-ups, antecedents, and how to respond when the behaviors to increase and decrease are observed. As also indicated in **Chapter 6**, the complete behavior support plan can be made available for staff trainees to review when they have the time to obtain background and related information regarding the plan.

Regardless of whether the **Behavior Support Plan Summary Form** or other type of checklist is used, it is important that each staff member receive a copy of the written summary of the procedures necessary to carry out a given consumer's support plan. Providing a written summary for each staff trainee is not a very common practice in many service settings. Rather, a copy of the support plan or some version thereof usually is placed in a central location in staffs' work area. It is recommend that a written summary be placed in staffs' routine work space *and* a copy be given to each staff member.

The rationale for providing a written summary of a behavior support plan in a central location as well as for each staff person is to adhere to a basic tenet of human behavior, including daily work performance of human service staff: *the easier it is for someone to do something that should be done, the more likely it is that the person will do it.* By providing staff with their own copy of the summary as well as by providing a centrally located copy, it is easier for staff to access the summary relative to providing the summary in only one of the two situations. This is particularly the case if the relatively common practice of providing a written summary only in a central location is followed. In the latter case, increased effort often is required of staff to go to the specific location to access the summary relative to if they have their own copy in a place they choose. Such effort can reduce the likelihood that some staff will review the summary when they need to review it.

Steps comprising a behavior support plan should be described to staff verbally and in written form

Step 3: Demonstrate the Target Skills Being Trained

Once staff trainees have been provided with a verbal and written description of the skills being trained, the next step in the training process is for the trainer to demonstrate the skills. It is important that all performance expectations related to the target skills be demonstrated. The demonstrations generally are most effective if provided in staffs' regular work area under conditions as similar as possible to what occurs during the usual work routine. This type of *on-the-job training* ensures that the skills are amenable for application during the conditions in which staff are expected to perform the skills.

An alternative means of demonstrating skills targeted during staff training is through role-play demonstrations. In role plays, the staff trainer (and if necessary, with the assistance of other personnel) act out how to perform the skills in a simulation situation. This type of demonstration often occurs in an inservice classroom or office meeting room and represents a *classroom-training* approach. Classroom training procedures frequently require less time for the overall training process than on-the-job training procedures. Classroom training can usually be conducted with a group of staff whereas on-the-job training typically must be conducted with one staff person at a time. However, classroom-training procedures do not ensure that the skills being trained can actually be performed by trainees as part of their typical work routine. Hence, whenever classroom-training approaches are used, there still must be some subsequent on-the-job components to ensure the training is effective (see discussion in later paragraphs).

Physically demonstrating the skills that staff trainees are expected to learn can be a powerful training procedure. Although verbal and written descriptions of target skills are helpful, many people have difficulty translating what they hear or read into practice. Being able to see what is to be done is often more helpful for staff to learn to perform the task themselves. Relatedly, some individuals will likely be unsure of what they should do when given only verbal and written instructions, but are reluctant to let the trainer know that they do not understand something. For example, some people are embarrassed to express their uncertainty, and especially in front of their peers who are also being trained. Providing a demonstration of the target skills is one means of reducing the uncertainty that some staff may experience.

In order for a trainer to effectively demonstrate target skills as part of the staff training process, it is necessary that the trainer know how to perform the skills that are expected to be trained to staff. Noting that staff trainers need to know how to perform what they are expected to train to staff may seem at first glance to be asserting the obvious—it appears as common sense that before someone can train others to perform a skill, the former individual must be able to perform the skill. Nonetheless, this situation occurs in many human service settings, and especially in regard to training staff how to implement behavior support plans.

A common example of the situation just noted occurs in community settings such as group homes. A contract psychologist writes a behavior support plan for one of the home's consumers and then gives the plan to the home manager (or faxes or e-mails the plan to the manager). The psychologist expects the home manager to read the plan and then train direct support staff how to implement the plan. However, the home manager may have questions about aspects of the plan or misinterpret what should be done with certain parts of the plan. Consequently, the home manager is not prepared to adequately demonstrate each component of the plan as part of the training process for staff.

Again, whoever is responsible for training staff must have competency in performing the skills that are to be trained. Otherwise, the training will inevitably be ineffective. In the situation just illustrated, if it is expected that the home manager will train staff how to implement the support plan, then it is incumbent on the psychologist to ensure that the manager is adequately trained such that the manager can demonstrate implementation of the plan proficiently.

Whoever is responsible for training staff how to implement a behavior support plan must be skilled in carrying out the plan him/herself

Step 4: Observe as Trainees Practice Performing Target Skills

Immediately after the trainer demonstrates the skills being trained to staff, trainees should be observed as they practice performing the skills themselves. Staff practice of the skills being trained is essentially the cornerstone of both competency- and performance-based training. As with the trainer's demonstration of the target skills, staffs' practice in performing the skills can occur on-the-job or in a classroom role-play situation.

When training staff how to implement a behavior support plan, it is usually advantageous if staff initially practice implementing the steps comprising the plan in a role-play process instead of on the job. If the initial practice demonstrations are conducted on the job with the consumer for whom the plan is developed, the consumer may be negatively affected by staffs' practice activities if the staff are not yet sufficiently skilled in carrying out the plan. In contrast, role-play practices can be repeated as necessary (see subsequent discussion of **Step 5** of the training process) without any negative effect on the consumer. Additionally, when staff have demonstrated proficiency in implementing components of a support plan in a role-play situation, only a brief amount of subsequent on-the-job training is usually needed for staff to adequately perform the steps when actually interacting with a consumer.

Having staff practice carrying out the skills that are being trained is a critical but often overlooked component in staff training endeavors. Nevertheless, staff practice *must* occur if the training is to be consistently effective. Staff practice of the target skills is necessary to ensure that staff have actually learned how to do what is being trained (again, see discussion of **Step 5** of the training process)

Including staff practice in demonstrating the target skills as part of the overall training process is also in accordance with *adult learning* principles. Principles of adult learning stress that staff training is likely to be most successful if staff take an active part in the training process. Providing staff with opportunities to practice target skills helps make staff active participants in the training.

Requiring staff to practice the target skills necessary to carry out a behavior support plan is also advantageous because the process frequently results in questions regarding likely situations that may occur when the support plan is actually implemented. Practicing implementation of a plan in a role-play situation tends to encourage staff to think about how a respective consumer may respond to the plan, and affords the trainer opportunities to respond to staff concern about what to do in those situations.

A final reason for including staff practice as part of the overall training process is that once staff actually begin the role-play activities, the process often becomes more enjoyable for the staff trainees. Many people find active participation in training such as by practicing target skills more enjoyable than just listening to a trainer explain what needs to be done. Making the training process more enjoyable can increase staffs' acceptance of the training as well as their acceptance of the behavior support plan in general. As noted previously, increasing staff acceptance of aspects of the behavior support plan process can add substantially to staffs' willingness to implement the plan.

Step 5: Provide Feedback to Staff Regarding Their Proficiency in Performing Each Skill

In some ways, the training step of having staff practice performing the skills being trained is only as good as the feedback that is provided after the practice activity. Feedback presented to a trainee is necessary to let the trainee know how well the target skills were performed. As such, feedback should be provided by the trainer immediately after the practice activity in a manner that lets the trainee know what was performed satisfactorily and as needed, what was not performed at a satisfactory level. If the trainee did not perform all aspects of the target skills proficiently, then the feedback should also specify what the trainee needs to do differently in order to improve the performance.

Earlier it was noted that for staff training to be effective, staff trainers must be well versed in the skills they are attempting to train. It is likewise critical that staff trainers be skilled in observing trainee performance and giving feedback in the manner just summarized. However, being able to demonstrate a skill and being able to observe someone else perform the skill and then provide evaluative feedback represent two different (though related) trainer skills. It should not be assumed that personnel charged with training staff how to implement behavior support plans necessarily have the skills to observe staff performance and give informative feedback. Rather, staff training personnel often need to be trained and experienced in observing performance and giving feedback. Additional discussion on the critical elements of giving useful feedback is provided in **Chapters 10** and **11**.

Step 6: Repeat Steps 3 - 5 Until Each Staff Trainee Demonstrates Proficiency in Performing Each Skill

The final step in the staff training process involves repeating the previous three steps (trainer demonstration of target skills, trainee practice, and provision of feedback). This step should be continued until each trainee proficiently demonstrates each skill being trained. The process of repeating the demonstration, practice, and feedback until proficiency is observed completes the competency- and performance-based requirements of the training; each trainee continues performing the skills being trained until competence is demonstrated.

It is usually easier from a trainer's perspective if **Step 6** occurs initially through role play. Once performance competence is demonstrated during role-play situations, then the process should occur in an on-the-job manner with each staff person. As with the role-play activities, the on-the-job practice with feedback should continue until each trainee demonstrates satisfactory application of the target skills in the actual work situation. When the staff trainer observes a given staff person perform the skills competently in the work place, then and only then can the trainer be assured that the training has been successful.

Staff training should never be considered finished until the staff trainer observes each trainee proficiently perform the skills being trained in the trainee's usual work place during routine work situations

Special Considerations When Training Staff to Implement Behavior Support Plans

Who Should Be Involved in the Training Process

An important decision when preparing to train staff to implement an individual's behavior support plan is who will conduct the training. Generally, involvement in programs for training staff in human service settings to implement support plans follows one of four models. Probably the most common model is one in which the person who developed the support plan, who is usually a psychologist, behavior analyst, behavior specialist, or in some cases a QMRP or QDDP, is expected to train the staff. Another common model is one in which the staffs' immediate supervisor such as a group home manager or workshop supervisor trains the staff. A third model, which is more common in larger agencies, is that a designated staff development or human resource person has the responsibility of training staff how to carry out behavior support plans. Finally, a fourth model involves training being conducted by a combination of the personnel just mentioned.

Which of the just noted models is used for training purposes usually depends on the organization and available resources of a given human service agency. However, to be most successful, the training approach should always involve at least two people. The first person is the clinician who developed the behavior support plan. The second person is the immediate supervisor of the staff.

The rationale for involving both the author of the plan and the staff supervisor in the training process is the same as that noted in **Chapter 2** regarding the shared responsibility for supervising staffs' day-to-day implementation of behavior support plans. To review briefly, the person who developed the plan should be involved in training staff because that person knows the most about what constitutes the plan. As such, the author of the plan is in the best position to accurately describe and demonstrate how the plan should be carried out. The plan's author is also usually in the best position to answer questions that staff may have concerning aspects of the plan. In regard to the supervisor's involvement in training staff, the supervisor is the person to whom staff are most likely to listen and respond in terms of successfully learning how to implement the plan.

In addition to obtaining staffs' attention in learning how to carry out a treatment plan, there are two other advantages of involving the supervisor in the staff training process. First, involvement in the training process helps to ensure that the supervisor is well versed in the knowledge and skills needed to implement a respective plan. Such information is critical in allowing the supervisor to support staff in carrying out their daily duties associated with implementing the plan. Second, and related to the first advantage, is that when staff are aware of their supervisor's knowledge and support of the plan—which becomes apparent when a supervisor takes the time to help train staff how to implement the plan—staff become more motivated to carry out the plan appropriately. As indicated in **Chapter 2** (see also discussion in **Chapters 10** and **11** related to supervising staffs' routine application of a treatment plan), staff usually are more likely to do things when requested or directed by their immediate supervisor than when requested or directed by clinicians or other agency personnel.

Both the staff supervisor and the author of an individual's behavior support plan should be involved in training staff how to carry out the plan with the individual

Which Staff Need to Be Trained to Carry Out Behavior Support Plans

If a behavior support plan is to successfully help an individual overcome one or more problem behaviors, all staff who interact with the individual must know how to carry out the plan. Consequently, when the plan is developed, all staff who interact with the individual will need to be trained regarding the plan's rationale and constituent procedures. Ensuring all staff are trained to competency in implementing a plan is critical to the plan's eventual success.

Making sure all staff receive competency- and performance-based training in carrying out a treatment plan can be a challenging process, and particularly in residential settings. Residential settings usually have several contingents of direct support staff who interact with each consumer and therefore, several groups of staff who need to be trained regarding a consumer's behavior plan. For instance, there may be day shift staff, afternoon/evening shift staff, and night shift staff. There may also be designated weekend staff and special relief staff (e.g., personnel who come in temporarily to cover for absent staff). Training each of these groups of staff can be a time- and labor-intensive process. Staff trainers must work with each group of staff for training purposes at the various times when the staff are routinely at work. In short, staff trainers will probably have to conduct a number of training sessions at different times in order to train every staff member.

In most cases, there is no alternative to spending time with each group of staff for training purposes. Unfortunately, the time- and labor-intensive features of the process are exacerbated by the fact that even staff comprising one particular group (e.g., evening shift staff) will work on different days. Hence, even for a given group, the staff trainers will need to meet with various staff at different times. The logistical problems that exist due to the different groups warranting training, and the different work schedules within each group, represent one reason training is frequently ineffective—trainers do not manage to train everybody who needs training. The end result is that some staff are working with a given consumer each week who are not skilled in carrying out the consumer's support plan.

The only way to avoid the situation in which some staff are not prepared to carry out a consumer's support plan is to make sure people responsible for training staff do indeed train every staff person who is expected to interact with the consumer. To possibly reduce the time and effort necessary to conduct the training, it is recommended that personnel who are expected to train staff make it readily apparent to agency executives just how much time is necessary for training purposes. Sometimes senior agency personnel are aware of the need for staff training in regard to preparing staff to implement support plans, but are not aware of the time commitment required of clinicians and supervisors to conduct the training in an effective manner.

Making sure agency executives are aware of the time commitment for necessary staff training can increase the likelihood that sufficient resources will be allocated for training purposes. Senior management may, for example, be able to designate certain personnel to assist with training on a part-time basis. Awareness among senior personnel regarding staff training needs can also be helpful in terms of generating more general support for training endeavors. To illustrate, a problem faced by many clinicians is that when sessions are scheduled to train staff in regard to carrying out a consumer's treatment plan, various staff fail to show up for the sessions. Increased time and effort is then required on the part of the clinician to arrange additional training sessions. If however, senior agency personnel openly and frequently espouse the importance of staff receiving training in treatment plan procedures, staffs' motivation to attend scheduled training sessions is likely to be enhanced. The beneficial effects of management support on the success of staff training endeavors is another example of how the prevention and treatment of challenging behavior should be an accepted responsibility of an agency's entire organization as discussed in the introductory comments to this text; successful prevention and treatment can rarely be accomplished by clinicians or front-line supervisors alone.

Placing Staff Training in the Proper Perspective for Ensuring Behavior Support Plans Are Carried Out Proficiently

Throughout this chapter, the importance of staff training has been stressed. Training staff how to implement behavior support plans is a critical step in the overall process of ensuring that the plans are carried out in the manner that they are intended to be carried out. However, it must be remembered that staff training is only one step in this process. Without the other component steps of outcome management, staff training is not likely to have a consistent impact on the day-to-day prevention and treatment of challenging behavior. In short, staff training is *a necessary but not sufficient step* in the overall process of implementing behavior support plans for challenging behavior.

In the overall process of ensuring behavior support plans are carried out in the appropriate manner, staff training is *a necessary but not sufficient step*

It is well established that training sets the occasion for desirable work performance among direct support staff, but does not in and of itself ensure such performance. When staff training is conducted in a competency- and performance-based manner as described in this chapter, then many staff will carry out respective treatment plans exactly in the manner the plans should be carried out. Other staff, though well-trained, probably will not perform so desirably. To ensure that all staff implement program plans in an appropriate and effective manner, the other steps of outcome management must be followed. Remaining chapters in this text describe what supervisors and authors of treatment plans should do to make sure that once staff are trained to implement a behavior support plan, they do indeed implement the plan appropriately, consistently, and effectively.

Section IV

Monitoring and Evaluating Staff Proficiency in Implementing Behavior Support Plans

CHAPTER 8

AVOIDING STAFF DISCONTENT WHEN MONITORING IMPLEMENTATION OF BEHAVIOR SUPPORT PLANS

A defining characteristic of an outcome management approach to operating human service agencies is a focus on outcomes. The entire process of providing supports and services begins with delineation of the outcomes that are desired to be attained by and for agency consumers. **Chapters 3** through **5**, for example, described outcomes associated with establishing congregate environments that are safe, responsive, and habilitative. Once important outcomes are identified, then the other component procedures of outcome management can be used to ensure the outcomes are attained in a timely fashion.

Another primary characteristic of outcome management is the importance placed on *monitoring* outcome attainment. Monitoring the degree to which desired outcomes are attained is the yardstick with which quality agencies determine how well they are fulfilling their intended mission. Data stemming from objective and reliable monitoring systems allow agency management to make informed decisions regarding when changes in agency operations are necessary versus when existing practices should be continued.

Sound monitoring systems are particularly important in regard to outcomes associated with staff implementation of behavior support plans. Specifically, the degree to which two important outcomes are attained warrants monitoring. The first outcome, which pertains to staff performance, is that staff consistently carry out treatment plans in the manner the plans are intended to be carried out. The second outcome concerns the behavior of the consumer recipients of the support plans. The desired outcome for consumers is improvement in the targeted problem behavior that support plans are designed to treat.

Monitoring Staff Implementation of Behavior Support Plans and Consumer Outcome Attainment

Systematically monitoring staff implementation of behavior support plans and the behavior of consumers is critical in the prevention and treatment of challenging behavior. Staff performance must be monitored to help ensure consumers receive supports and services dictated by treatment plans designed to overcome challenging behavior (i.e., to help ensure staff perform in a manner that provides the desired treatment services). Consumer behavior must be monitored to ensure that the treatment plans are effective when appropriately carried out.

When there is no systematic monitoring of the implementation and effectiveness of behavior support plans, treatment attempts usually become inconsistent and ineffective. A common scenario in many congregate settings is that agency personnel become disgruntled with a given support plan because the consumer for whom the plan was designed continues to display problem behavior. In many cases though, disgruntlement concerning ineffectiveness of the support plan is not warranted because the plan is not adequately implemented by respective staff. Without information from a monitoring system regarding how well staff implement the plan, there is no way for agency personnel to know that the plan could be effective but that staff are not carrying out the plan appropriately. The usual result is that changes are made in the program procedures in an attempt to reduce the problem behavior more effectively. However, when the changes are made, there is no way to accurately evaluate the effects of each change because there is no objective monitoring of how well staff implement the changes, or how the consumer responds to each change. In short, the treatment attempts represent little more than guess work, and rarely attain the desired outcomes.

The situation just illustrated presents numerous problems for both people with severe disabilities and human service staff. For people with severe disabilities, they do not benefit from the existing technology for understanding and treating challenging behavior. When agency personnel make frequent changes in how they respond to problem behavior in the manner just described, the changes are rarely based on an empirically substantiated means of preventing and treating challenging behavior. Rather, the changes often are based on immediate impulse, guess work, or desperation. Whereas intervention procedures based on an empirically and socially validated technology (see **Chapter 6**) usually result in successful prevention and treatment of problem behavior, procedures based on impulse, guess work, or desperation rarely help people overcome challenging behavior.

Support plans for challenging behavior are rarely effective if there is not systematic monitoring of staff implementation of the plans and consumer response to the plans

From the perspective of direct service staff, the impact of attempting to treat challenging behavior without information stemming from a sound monitoring system is detrimental in several ways. In particular, when staff are repeatedly expected to change how they work with a given consumer who has problem behavior because each preceding treatment approach was ineffective, staff become frustrated. As each treatment attempt fails, staff become less optimistic about new treatment approaches. Staff also lose faith in agency clinicians and related personnel who repeatedly change treatment procedures but achieve little success in decreasing a consumer's problem behavior. Because direct service staff must deal with the problem behavior on a frequent basis, they often resort to their own means of attempting to prevent or respond to the problem behavior when they believe formal support plans are not effective. In many cases, staffs' informal or impromptu treatment attempts—although well intended—tend to exacerbate the problem. In the most extreme cases, staff reliance on informal and impromptu approaches to challenging behavior lead to consumer abuse or neglect.

The situations just illustrated reflect the importance of monitoring in the prevention and treatment of challenging behavior, and what can happen when monitoring is not a part of the support plan process. Because of the recognized importance of routine monitoring, many human service agencies regularly monitor staff performance associated with carrying out behavior support plans. Unfortunately though, a considerable number of these agencies have experienced serious problems in their attempts to monitor staff work performance.

Problems with monitoring systems experienced by human service agencies have resulted in a frequent dislike of monitoring among both management and staff. However, the problems are not inherent in the practice of monitoring per se, but due to: (1) how monitoring is performed and, (2) how the results of monitoring are used within an agency. In this regard, there are a number of human service agencies that routinely monitor staff implementation of behavior support plans without any significant problems. The success of the latter agencies in systematically monitoring staff performance as part of the support plan process is strong evidence that monitoring in and of itself does not have to be problematic.

The purpose of this chapter is to describe the most frequent problems that arise with performance monitoring systems in congregate settings, and how those problems can be avoided. By following several key procedural guidelines, monitoring can be conducted in a way that not only enhances the prevention and treatment of challenging behavior among agency consumers, but also improves the quality of staffs' work environment from a job satisfaction perspective. Following discussion of how monitoring can be conducted in an effective and acceptable manner, **Chapter 9** describes a specific monitoring system that can be used to obtain relevant information about staff implementation of behavior support plans.

Avoiding Common Problems in the Way Staff Implementation of Behavior Support Plans is Monitored

Most problems associated with monitoring systems designed to obtain information about staff work behavior are related to one factor: staff in human service agencies usually do not like other agency personnel monitoring their work performance. When staff become aware that someone, and particularly a management representative, will be monitoring their work activities, the reaction engendered among staff is usually not very positive. When the person assigned to do the monitoring actually arrives at the work site to observe staff performance, the reactions among staff are usually even less positive.

When staff seriously dislike a management practice, the practice is often terminated or conducted in an incomplete fashion that seriously reduces the utility of the practice. In the case of monitoring work performance, staff often complain about the practice to their supervisors as well as whoever is conducting the monitoring. Anyone who has had the responsibility of formally monitoring staff work performance has likely experienced negative reactions from the staff whose performance was being monitored. Such reactions cause agency personnel who are expected to perform the monitoring to avoid doing the monitoring if possible, or to do it in a hurried or incomplete manner.

Discontent with ongoing monitoring practices also impacts agency executives. As senior management personnel repeatedly hear concerns about ongoing monitoring practices, they tend to discontinue the practices—monitoring comes to be viewed as causing more problems than it solves. When monitoring of staff performance is discontinued due to negative reactions among staff, or monitoring begins to occur in an inadequate manner, a key component of effective supervision is lost. Monitoring staff implementation of behavior support plans is the *only* way to truly know how well or poorly the plans are being carried out. Hence, it is necessary to find ways to monitor staff performance without causing staff disgruntlement.

As noted earlier, some agencies routinely monitor staff performance associated with carrying out behavior support plans with minimal or no signs of staff displeasure. In a number of these agencies, staff actually look forward to having their work duties observed by others. The difference in reactions to performance monitoring in these agencies relative to agencies in which monitoring procedures have resulted in staff disgruntlement is *how* and *why* the monitoring is conducted.

There are four common ways in which monitoring is conducted in human service agencies that result in staff discontent with the monitoring. These ways are summarized below. When these particular monitoring practices are avoided, negative reactions among staff to performance monitoring are greatly reduced or prevented altogether.

WAYS IN WHICH MONITORING IS CONDUCTED THAT RESULT IN NEGATIVE STAFF REACTIONS TO THE MONITORING

1) Attempts are made to monitor staff performance covertly

2) Staff are not informed of the purpose of the monitoring

3) Monitoring occurs in an impolite or rude manner

4) Results of the monitoring are not readily shared with staff

Monitoring Should Always Be Overt

For the type of monitoring discussed here—that is, monitoring staff proficiency in implementing behavior support plans—the monitoring should always be conducted in an open or *overt* manner. People responsible for designing and implementing monitoring systems for use with staff work performance should always make sure that staff know their performance will be monitored. Attempting to monitor staff performance without staff awareness of the monitoring, or *covert* monitoring, should be avoided.

Using covert means to monitor staff work performance almost always causes serious problems. In typical human service agencies the monitoring rarely remains covert. Staff invariably become aware that someone in the agency is monitoring their work performance. When staff realize that someone is attempting to observe their performance in a secretive manner, they usually become most displeased with the monitoring. Covert monitoring results in a feeling of distrust toward people responsible for the monitoring as well as agency management in general. A "we versus them" attitude develops that is highly detrimental for the overall operation of the agency and ultimately, for the quality of supports and services provided to agency consumers.

Not only should covert monitoring be avoided because of staff disgruntlement that monitoring causes, there is essentially no good reason to monitor in a secretive manner. The purpose of monitoring as represented here is to assess how staff are carrying out program plans for challenging behavior and either help staff change certain procedures if necessary, or explicitly support staff in continuing to implement the plans correctly. Monitoring also allows an opportunity to see how a respective consumer is responding to various aspects of a treatment plan. As such, staff should be informed early in the treatment planning process that monitoring to determine how the plan is working and how a consumer is responding to the plan is a regular component of treatment activities. As indicated in the next section, when staff know beforehand that a supervisor or author of a support plan intends to observe the plan in action, and the person then routinely visits staffs' work area to observe the plan, they are often appreciative of the person's efforts to help make the plan effective.

Staff Should Be Aware of the Specific Purpose of Monitoring

When staff are aware that someone such as a supervisor or clinician will be visiting their work site to observe implementation of a behavior support plan, then staff know what the person is doing when the individual arrives at the work site for monitoring purposes. Staff are likewise aware of the reason for the monitoring. This approach to monitoring is much different than what occurs in a number of cases in which staff are aware that their work activities are being observed (i.e., the monitoring is overt) but are not exactly sure what is being observed or why. When staff know they are being observed but do not know precisely what is being observed or the purpose of the monitoring, staff usually become anxious or otherwise concerned about the observations.

Staff anxiety about having their performance observed usually occurs because of negative experiences staff have had with previous monitoring practices. In many human service agencies, monitoring is primarily conducted when something undesirable has occurred in the agency. Managers begin monitoring in order to determine who is responsible for certain problems that have occurred, and to prevent such activities from being repeated. The monitoring is frequently followed by negative sanctions directed toward certain staff, such as negative feedback or disciplinary action. When monitoring has occurred for these reasons and staff become aware that their work is being formally monitored, they begin to expect that something undesirable will follow the monitoring. Monitoring serves as a signal that negative management action is forthcoming.

Negative reactions among staff to having their performance observed also occur because of other experiences with agency monitoring procedures. Many agencies tend to monitor certain staff activities only when the agencies are expecting some type of external evaluation, such as the Title XIX ICF-MR Medicaid surveys conducted in a number of congregate residential settings. When agency management expects a survey to be pending, agency representatives begin to monitor staff activities in an attempt to prepare for the survey and avoid problem situations that the survey may encounter. Although this practice may have merit from an overall agency perspective in terms of preparing for the survey, the impact on direct support staff is often quite negative. Experienced staff become aware that their performance, such as that associated with implementation of behavior support plans, is only of concern to agency management when a survey is expected. Staff view monitoring in these situations as only serving management's interests, and not as representing true concern for their work with consumers who display problem behavior. The end result is a feeling of disrespect or mistrust of agency management.

When routine monitoring of staff performance occurs as a means to help program plans serve the intended purpose of overcoming challenging behavior, the purpose of the monitoring is much different than that reflected in the situations just illustrated. The intent is to make sure the plans are implemented appropriately and effectively, and staff are provided sufficient information, training, and support to carry out their duties proficiently. Because direct service staff are usually most interested in reducing challenging behavior among consumers with whom they work, observations conducted for the latter purpose are often welcomed or at the least, not perceived as an unpleasant event.

Staff should be well informed that routine monitoring of the implementation of behavior support plans is a critical component in the overall prevention and treatment of challenging behavior

Practicing Common Courtesy When Monitoring Staff Implementation of Behavior Support Plans

Much of the staff disgruntlement that accompanies traditional ways in which monitoring is conducted can be avoided if monitors practice common courtesy when observing staff work performance. Common courtesy should of course accompany any management practice in the human services. Because of the negative impact that performance monitoring often has on the people being observed though, common courtesy is especially important when monitoring staff work activities.

Noting the importance of common courtesy may appear at first glance to be asserting the obvious. However, the way staff work performance is frequently monitored in human service agencies suggests that courteous practices are not a routine occurrence. To illustrate, many monitors enter a staff work station and begin their monitoring duties without greeting or otherwise acknowledging the staff who are present. In typical social situations, when someone enters a room with other people present and essentially ignores everyone, the behavior appears impolite or rude. The same effect results when monitors begin their observations of staff without greeting or saying anything to the staff.

In defense of agency personnel charged with staff monitoring duties, often the failure to acknowledge staff is because monitors do not want to interfere with staff work activities. In other cases, monitors simply want to conduct the monitoring expeditiously, and exit staffs' work area as quickly as possible. The latter situation typically occurs because monitors have experienced negative staff reactions to past efforts to monitor staff work duties. Nonetheless, the impact of the process on staff perception of the monitoring is quite negative.

To avoid unpleasantness for staff that accompanies the beginning of a monitoring process as just illustrated, monitors should always greet staff upon entering their work station. The greeting should occur just as it would normally happen in typical social situations in which a person enters a room with other people present. Following the initial greeting, it is likewise helpful if the monitor informs staff that the purpose of the monitoring is to see how the support plan process is going with a given consumer's challenging behavior, and how the consumer reacts to staffs' implementation of the plan. This quick gesture, though simple in nature, can go a long way toward enhancing staff acceptance of the monitoring process, as well as the monitor.

Another common situation reflecting lack of common courtesy is when a monitor leaves staffs' work area after completing the monitoring without saying anything to staff. Many monitors fail to extend this common social gesture because they are in a hurry to proceed with their other duties, or they simply want to avoid interacting with staff. The latter situation occurs because again, monitors have had negative experiences with staff reactions to having their performance monitored. Either way, the process is at least awkward for staff and at worst, very unpleasant.

Monitors should take the few minutes of time necessary to acknowledge to staff that they have finished their monitoring and will be leaving the area. This is another simple gesture that can have a significant impact on staff acceptance of the monitoring and the monitor. As described in the next section, it can also be very useful if monitors provide feedback to staff about the monitoring before leaving the immediate area.

Provide Staff With Feedback as Quickly as Possible Once Monitoring is Completed

When monitors leave staffs' work station without any interaction with staff, there is a detrimental impact on staff acceptance of the monitoring beyond the effects of being discourteous. Staff are usually interested in the results of the monitoring of their performance. When monitors leave without interacting with staff, there is no opportunity for staff to learn about the outcome of the monitoring.

When staff are aware that someone is formally monitoring their work performance, often they experience a certain degree of anxiety concerning what the monitor observed and the corresponding evaluation of their work performance. If a monitor takes the time to explain to staff what was observed and what it means, the anxiety is typically reduced or eliminated. Reducing or eliminating staff anxiety makes the monitoring process less unpleasant for staff relative to the situation in which anxiety persists because the monitor does not inform staff about the outcome of the monitoring.

Providing information, or feedback, to staff about the results of monitoring has an important impact in addition to enhancing staff acceptance of the monitoring. As noted earlier, the purpose of monitoring in this situation is to obtain first-hand information about how a plan is being implemented and how the consumer is responding to various aspects of the plan. Information obtained during the monitoring can be used to help change what staff are doing with the plan if changes are warranted, or explicitly support staff in continuing to implement the plan in their current manner. If information is not provided to staff following the monitoring, then neither of the latter two functions can be achieved.

In short, the purpose of monitoring is to help staff improve their implementation of a behavior support plan or to reinforce their ongoing efforts. For monitoring to serve these purposes, monitors must provide feedback to staff regarding their observed performance. Unless such feedback is provided, there is little reason to monitor staff performance. Detailed information on the importance of feedback and how it should be presented to staff is provided in **Chapters 10** and **11**.

KEYS TO ENHANCING STAFF ACCEPTANCE OF HAVING THEIR PERFORMANCE MONITORED WHEN IMPLEMENTING SUPPORT PLANS

1. **Ensure staff are aware that their performance will be observed; never conduct observations in a secretive manner**
2. **Inform staff of the specific purpose of the monitoring**
3. **Use common courtesy when conducting observations; interact with staff when entering and leaving staffs' work area**
4. **Provide feedback to staff as soon as possible once the monitoring is completed**

Avoiding Problems With How Results of Monitoring Are Used

If the procedures just summarized are followed, many of the concerns with how staff respond to having their performance monitored will be alleviated. However, not all of the reasons staff tend to dislike performance monitoring will be addressed. Attention also needs to be directed to how results of the monitoring are used by agency management.

There are two guidelines management should follow in using information that results from monitoring staff implementation of behavior support plans to help make monitoring acceptable to staff. The first guideline was just noted when considering how monitoring is conducted: *monitors should provide feedback to staff about results of the monitoring as soon as possible after completing the observations.* Management should design the entire monitoring process such that information stemming from the monitoring can be given to staff in a timely manner. In many human service agencies, monitoring systems are designed such that feedback to staff is likely to be significantly delayed.

A number of human service agencies include monitoring staffs' implementation of behavior support plans as part of an overall quality assurance or improvement system that involves monitoring a number of an agency's operations. Typically, these systems involve certain personnel who have the designated responsibility of routinely monitoring and collecting data on aspects of staff work performance. The monitoring data are forwarded to a central office for summary and analysis. A report is then prepared and sent to agency management on a weekly, monthly, or quarterly basis. In turn, management reviews and distributes the report through the agency's organizational chain of command.

Quality assurance or improvement systems as just described can be valuable tools for operating human service agencies in an efficient and effective manner. However, from the perspective of providing timely feedback to staff regarding observations of their performance, the systems are of little value. If monitoring data are collected and distributed in the manner just summarized, information about the monitoring reaches staff long after their work performance has been observed. Even if management reviews and distributes the information on a weekly basis, by the time the information filters through the chain of command and goes from staffs' immediate supervisor to staff, a lengthy delay has occurred since staff were observed. The end result is the undesirable situation described earlier in which staff are left wondering about the outcome of the observations of their work performance.

To avoid the delay in providing feedback to staff based on observations of their performance, quality assurance systems should be designed such that monitors give feedback to staff immediately after observing staff performance. The information can still be processed through the overall summary and review system just noted in terms of preparation and distribution of periodic reports. In this way, the information can be used by management for larger-scale, quality assurance purposes but staff are not required to wait lengthy time periods to be informed of results of the monitoring.

A second guideline regarding how management should use information resulting from monitoring in terms of enhancing staff acceptance of the monitoring is to *focus on the positive aspects of observed performance.* There is a common management tendency to look for things that are going wrong within an agency and then provide negative sanctions to the responsible staff. In regard to using results of monitoring systems, management tends to focus on the *negative* aspects of staffs' work performance. Management focus on what is wrong with staff performance is a primary reason that staff have had negative experiences with monitoring and why staff dislike monitoring systems in general.

Reasons why management in various human service agencies tends to focus on identifying and responding to problems with staff performance in contrast to taking a more positive, supportive stance is beyond the scope of this chapter. The last two chapters in this manual discuss in detail how an outcome management approach can be used by agency supervisors and clinicians to take a more supportive and positive approach to operating human service agencies, while still correcting areas of staff performance that warrant improvement. The point here is that management should refrain from focusing on negative aspects of staff performance in regard to staff implementation of behavior support plans. The emphasis should be on recognizing and commending appropriate staff performance. Relatedly, the focus should be on providing adequate specification of duties, performance- and competency-based training of staff, and provision of adequate resources as described in previous chapters that make it likely staff will carry out behavior support plans in an acceptable manner. If the previously described component steps of outcome management are followed in regard to preparing staff to implement behavior support plans, then problems with staff implementation will be the exception rather than the rule. When problems do occur, corrective management procedures (**Chapter 11**) can then be implemented to resolve the problems.

A Final Note On the Importance of Routinely Monitoring Staff Implementation of Behavior Support Plans

In **Chapter 7** it was stressed that effective staff training is an integral part of an outcome management approach for preventing and treating challenging behavior. It was also emphasized that staff training is only one of several key steps for ensuring staff perform their work duties in a way to effectively prevent or reduce consumer problem behavior. Monitoring staff work duties as discussed in this chapter represents a similar process in terms of its component role within outcome management.

Like staff training, monitoring of staff work performance is a *necessary but not sufficient* step for ensuring effective prevention and treatment of challenging behavior. Performance monitoring must be performed in conjunction with the steps of outcome management described in preceding chapters. Likewise, performance monitoring must be accompanied by the steps to be discussed in **Chapters 10** and **11** on supportive and corrective management, respectively. Nonetheless, monitoring of staff work duties associated with carrying out behavior support plans is a critical part of outcome management. The next chapter describes a specific means of objectively and accurately monitoring staff performance associated with behavior support plan implementation. If the monitoring procedures described in the next chapter are employed in conjunction with the guidelines described here, then not only will the prevention and treatment of challenging behavior be enhanced, but staff acceptance of the entire process will be maximized.

CHAPTER 9

A Specific Process for Monitoring Staff Implementation of Behavior Support Plans

Chapter 8 described the importance of routinely monitoring staff implementation of support plans for challenging behavior. To review briefly, systematic monitoring of the way staff carry out behavior support plans is the only means of knowing that the plans are being implemented in the appropriate and prescribed manner. Information that results from monitoring also allows supervisors and authors of treatment plans to actively support staff in continuing to carry out their implementation duties proficiently, as well as to correct staff performance when implementation is not adequate.

Guidelines for Monitoring Implementation of Behavior Support Plans in a Manner Acceptable to Staff

1. **Ensure staff are aware that their performance will be monitored**
2. **Inform staff of the specific purpose of the monitoring**
3. **Use common courtesy when monitoring; interact with staff when entering and leaving their work area**
4. **Provide feedback to staff as quickly as possible after completing the monitoring**

Chapter 8 likewise presented guidelines for monitoring implementation of behavior support plans in a way that is generally well received by staff. The essence of conducting a monitoring session in a manner acceptable to staff—and in a way that avoids staff disgruntlement that typically accompanies traditional ways in which performance monitoring is conducted—is summarized above.

This chapter continues the focus on monitoring staff implementation of support plans for challenging behavior. More precisely, the purpose is to describe a specific means of monitoring the proficiency with which staff carry out behavior support plans. The process to be described has been used in a number of congregate settings to objectively observe how well staff implement a wide variety of support plans. The process is designed to be applicable with essentially any type of behavior support plan that direct service staff would be expected to implement with individuals who have severe disabilities and challenging behavior. The process also is designed to be used in accordance with the just noted guidelines for monitoring staff performance in a way that is likely to be well received by direct support personnel.

Steps for Monitoring Staff Implementation of Behavior Support Plans

A prerequisite to monitoring the proficiency with which staff carry out a behavior support plan is knowing what staff are suppose to do to implement the plan's procedures. Hence, the first step in monitoring staff performance is to review the written plan to identify each specific procedure that staff should implement. As discussed in **Chapter 6**, this step is facilitated if a form such as the **Behavior Support Plan Summary Form** is used (see following illustration for review).

Behavior Support Plan Summary Form

Consumer name:________________ Date plan begins:________

Target Behaviors

What are the behaviors to decrease?

What are the behaviors to increase?

Environmental Set-ups

What should be present in the everyday environment?

What should not be present in the everyday environment?

Antecedents

What event often happens right before a problem behavior?

What should be done if the event happens?

Consequences

What should be done if the behavior to decrease occurs?

What should be done if the behavior to increase occurs?

Figure 9-1: *Behavior Support Plan Summary Form* (see Chapter 6 for discussion)

The **Behavior Support Plan Summary Form** categorizes the procedures that constitute behavior support plans into: (1) *target behaviors* (behaviors to increase and decrease), (2) *environmental set-ups* (what should and should not be in place in the consumer's environment), (3) *antecedents* (what tends to occur immediately before the consumer displays the problem behavior and what staff should do when the antecedents are observed) and, (4) what staff should do in response to the behaviors to increase and decrease, or the desired *consequences* to the behaviors.

If the **Behavior Support Plan Summary Form** or a similar instrument is completed by answering the questions on the form, it should be readily apparent what staff are expected to do to implement a support plan. Correspondingly, it should be readily apparent what the observer should expect to see staff do when observing staffs' implementation of the plan.

In order to obtain accurate information about how well or poorly staff implement each part of a behavior support plan, monitoring of their implementation must occur in a consistent manner. If monitoring is not performed consistently, it is impossible to obtain an accurate picture of staff implementation proficiency over time; differences in information obtained from one monitoring session to another are likely to be due to differences in how the monitoring is performed and not necessarily to how staff are actually carrying out the plan.

Consistency in monitoring staff performance can be enhanced if a designated observation form is used to conduct each monitoring session. The **Behavior Support Plan Implementation Monitoring Form** provided in the following illustration was developed specifically for maintaining consistency when observing staff carry out a behavior support plan (see also the **Appendix** for a copy of the form). The **Monitoring Form** is designed in accordance with the four basic categories of behavior support plans. The following chapter sections describe the steps monitors should follow when using the **Behavior Support Plan Implementation Monitoring Form** to observe staff performance when staff are expected to carry out behavior support plans.

Behavior Support Plan Implementation Monitoring Form

Consumer ________ **Location** ________ **Activity** ______________

Staff present ______________ **Date** ______ **Time** ______ **Observer** ________

Environmental Set-ups

Antecedents

Behaviors to increase

Staff response to behaviors to increase

Behaviors to decrease

Staff responses to behaviors to decrease

Env. S-U	Antecedents	Beh. to Increase	Staff Response	Beh. to Decrease	Staff Response
1. Y N NA	Y N NA	Y N NA	Y N NA	Y N NA	Y N NA
2. Y N NA	Y N NA	Y N NA	Y N NA	Y N NA	Y N NA
3. Y N NA	Y N NA	Y N NA	Y N NA	Y N NA	Y N NA
4. Y N NA	Y N NA	Y N NA	Y N NA	Y N NA	Y N NA
5. Y N NA	Y N NA	Y N NA	Y N NA	Y N NA	Y N NA
6. Y N NA	Y N NA	Y N NA	Y N NA	Y N NA	Y N NA
7. Y N NA	Y N NA	Y N NA	Y N NA	Y N NA	Y N NA
8. Y N NA	Y N NA	Y N NA	Y N NA	Y N NA	Y N NA
9. Y N NA	Y N NA	Y N NA	Y N NA	Y N NA	Y N NA
10. Y N NA	Y N NA	Y N NA	Y N NA	Y N NA	Y N NA
#Y / #Y+N = ___	#Y / #Y+N= ___		#Y / #Y+N = ___		#Y / #Y+N= ___
%Y ___	%Y ___		%Y ___		%Y ___

Total #Y / #Y+N= ______ Overall % Y ______

Figure 9-2: *Behavior Support Plan Implementation Monitoring Form* for observing and evaluating staff implementation of a behavior support plan for an individual's challenging behavior.

Preparing the Monitoring Form Prior to Monitoring

Prior to conducting a monitoring session regarding staff implementation of a consumer's support plan, basic identifying information should be written on the top of the monitoring form. This information identifies the consumer who is to be observed, the location of the observation, the activity that is ongoing when the observation is initiated, which staff are present, the date and time of the observation, and who is conducting the observation. Next, information from the behavior support plan (or from the **Behavior Support Plan Summary Form**) pertaining to necessary procedures to carry out the plan should be written on the form. The headings in the box on the upper portion of the monitoring form relate to the basic categories of behavior support plan procedures: *environmental set-ups, antecedents, behaviors to increase* (along with *staff responses to the behaviors to increase*), and *behaviors to decrease* (and respective *staff responses*). Critical information for implementing the support plan associated with each of these categories should be transcribed onto the monitoring form.

The following illustration shows how the top portion of the monitoring form has been completed with information from the behavior support plan for an individual (Patti) who resides in a group home. Subsequent paragraphs provide more detail about the kinds of information that should be listed under each of the designated headings.

Environmental Set-ups to Prevent the Occurrence of Problem Behavior

As noted previously, whenever possible support plans should include information about environmental conditions that set the occasion for the occurrence of problem behavior, as well as conditions that reduce the likelihood that problem behavior will occur. Exactly what staff should do to arrange the environment to

Behavior Support Plan Implementation Monitoring Form

Consumer *Patti* Location *group home* Activity *leisure*

Staff present *Stan, Beth* Date *1/15/02* Time *5:30* Observer *Becklum*

Environmental Set-ups *during leisure times, Patti should have leisure materials in arms reach; she should not be in a room with her peers unless a staff person is present*

Antecedents
repeatedly saying the same thing; when she does this, she should be prompted to engage with materials (usually her video game)

Behaviors to increase
manipulating leisure materials

Staff response to behaviors to increase
give her attention (e.g., sit next to her) as much as possible; must praise or talk to her at least every 5 minutes

Behaviors to decrease
pulling on the clothing of her peers

Staff responses to behaviors to decrease
interrupt the pulling, escort her away from the peer and prompt her to engage with the leisure materials

Env. S-U	Antecedents	Beh. to Increase	Staff Response	Beh. to Decrease	Staff Response
1. Y N NA	Y N NA	Y N NA	Y N NA	Y N NA	Y N NA
2. Y N NA	Y N NA	Y N NA	Y N NA	Y N NA	Y N NA
3. Y N NA	Y N NA	Y N NA	Y N NA	Y N NA	Y N NA
4. Y N NA	Y N NA	Y N NA	Y N NA	Y N NA	Y N NA
5. Y N NA	Y N NA	Y N NA	Y N NA	Y N NA	Y N NA
6. Y N NA	Y N NA	Y N NA	Y N NA	Y N NA	Y N NA
7. Y N NA	Y N NA	Y N NA	Y N NA	Y N NA	Y N NA
8. Y N NA	Y N NA	Y N NA	Y N NA	Y N NA	Y N NA
9. Y N NA	Y N NA	Y N NA	Y N NA	Y N NA	Y N NA
10. Y N NA	Y N NA	Y N NA	Y N NA	Y N NA	Y N NA
#Y / #Y+N = ___	#Y / #Y+N = ___		#Y / #Y+N = ___		#Y / #Y+N = ___
%Y ___	%Y ___		%Y ___		%Y ___

Total #Y / #Y+N = ______ Overall % Y ______

Figure 9-3: *Sample Behavior Support Plan Implementation Monitoring Form* with information filled in regarding what to look for when observing staff implementation of an individual's (Patti) behavior support plan.

support the occurrence of adaptive behavior and minimize the occurrence of problem behavior should be described. More precisely, what should and should not be present in the consumer's immediate environment should be denoted on the **Behavior Support Plan Implementation Monitoring Form**. For the support plan represented on the form just illustrated for example, Patti (the consumer) should have leisure materials within arm's reach during leisure times and she should not be in a room with any of her peers without a staff person present in the room.

Antecedents

The antecedent section should be completed by specifying what often happens right before a problem behavior occurs. Equally importantly, what staff should do when the antecedent event happens should be specified. The intent is for staff to change what is ongoing as part of the antecedent in an attempt to prevent the problem behavior. If the antecedent event can be changed by staff once it begins, then the likelihood of the event leading to the problem behavior is reduced. To illustrate, on the form to monitor implementation of Patti's support plan, the antecedent to her behavior of pulling on the clothing of one of her peers in the group home (which occasions the peer becoming aggressive with Patti) is Patti engaging in repetitious speech. When she begins to say the same thing repeatedly, staff should prompt her to interact with the leisure materials that are present (e.g., her video game).

Consumer Behaviors to Increase

An important strategy discussed in preceding chapters for reducing problem behavior is to teach or increase socially acceptable behaviors that replace the need for a consumer to display problem behavior. To review, a consumer may engage in aggression, for example, in order to leave or escape an ongoing activity that the consumer does not enjoy. Aggression may be reduced in this situation by teaching the consumer a more socially acceptable way of asking to leave the activity such as by manually signing "stop". Producing the manual sign for "stop" when ready to end an activity would be a socially acceptable behavior that can serve the same function that aggression served for the consumer. Hence, signing "stop" instead of engaging in problem behavior represents a behavior to increase because of the reductive effect the manual signing could have on problem behavior.

In some cases, the function of a problem behavior is unclear, or it may take a considerable amount of time to teach a socially acceptable behavior to replace the need for the problem behavior. In these cases, behaviors that are incompatible with the problem behavior may be targeted to increase. To illustrate, if a consumer engages in self-injurious face slapping or head hitting, participation in activities that require using the hands in constructive ways may be behaviors to increase, such as playing a computer game, drawing, or working on a manipulative work task. In the illustration regarding implementation of Patti's behavior support plan, the behavior to increase is manipulating leisure materials.

Staff Response to Behaviors to Increase

What staff should do when the consumer engages in a behavior to be increased should be listed on the monitoring form under the designated heading. This information usually includes items or activities which should be provided as reinforcers. The category should also include information about how often reinforcers should be presented. For Patti's support plan, it is specified that staff should give her as much attention as possible (such as by sitting next to her) when she is manipulating leisure materials but at the least, talk to her or praise her at least once every five minutes while she is using the materials.

Consumer Behaviors to Decrease

The behavior to decrease, or problem behavior, should be described in sufficient detail so that staff can readily determine when the problem behavior occurs. Listing problem behavior in generic classes such as disruption, self-injury, or tantrums may not provide a sufficient description. Rather, staff usually need to know the specific behaviors of concern. To illustrate, rather than noting aggression as a behavior to decrease, specific behaviors such as hitting, kicking, biting, or slapping might be listed. If there is more than one problem behavior and staff must respond differently to each behavior, each problem behavior to which staff should respond in a certain way should be identified. With Patti's support plan, there is only one identified behavior to decrease, that of pulling on the clothes of her peers.

Staff Response to Behaviors to Decrease

The final category on the monitoring form is for listing how staff should respond when a problem behavior occurs. Staff response to each respective problem behavior should be clearly identified. Again referring to Patti's illustrated support plan, the desired staff response to Patti's targeted behavior to decrease (pulling on her peer's clothing) is to interrupt the pulling, escort her away from the peer, and prompt her to engage with the leisure materials that are present.

Conducting a Monitoring Session

Once the **Behavior Support Plan Implementation Monitoring Form** has been prepared with a summary of how the support plan should be implemented, the observer is ready to conduct an observation. Typically, one monitoring session requires 10 minutes. The 10-minute observation time is divided into 1-minute intervals for recording purposes. Initially, the observer watches the consumer and any staff who interact with the consumer during the first minute of the observation. After one minute of observation, the observer records what was observed regarding each category of the behavior support plan by marking the relevant category codes along the row of codes marked as "1" on the monitoring form. The observer can take up to 15 seconds to mark the observation form after each 1-minute of observation. The definitions corresponding to the category codes on the monitoring form are as follows.

Category Codes and Definitions for Using the Behavior Support Plan Implementation Monitoring Form

Environmental Set-Ups

Y (yes)—all things that should be present in the environment are observed *and* all things that should not be present are observed to be absent

N (no)—anything that should be present is absent *or* anything that should not be present is observed in the environment

NA (not applicable)—nothing was identified in the support plan that should be present or absent

Antecedents

Y (yes)—at least one identified antecedent was observed to occur, and staff responded appropriately to every antecedent event observed

N (no)—an identified antecedent was observed to occur and staff did not respond to the antecedent as dictated in the behavior support plan

NA (not applicable)—no antecedents to the problem behavior were observed to occur or no antecedents were identified in the behavior support plan

Behaviors to Increase

Y (yes)—*any* behavior to increase was observed to occur

N (no)—no behavior to increase was observed to occur

NA (not applicable)—no behavior to increase was identified in the behavior support plan

Staff Response to Behaviors to Increase

Y (yes)—staff responded in the designated manner to *every* behavior to increase that was observed to occur

N (no)—staff did not respond in the designated manner to a behavior to increase that was observed to occur

NA (not applicable)—no behavior to increase was observed to occur or behavior to increase was not identified in the behavior support plan

Behaviors to Decrease

Y (yes)—*any* behavior to decrease was observed to occur

N (no)—no behavior to decrease was observed to occur

NA (not applicable)—no behavior to decrease was identified in the behavior support plan

Staff Response to Behavior to Decrease

Y (yes)—staff responded in the designated manner to *every* behavior to decrease observed to occur

N (no)—staff did not respond in the designated manner to a behavior to decrease observed to occur

NA (not applicable)—no behavior to decrease was observed to occur or there was no behavior to decrease identified in the behavior support plan

After scoring the first minute on the monitoring form, the observer watches again for one minute and subsequently marks the relevant codes in each category along the second row of codes on the monitoring form. One minute of observation followed by scoring the corresponding row on the monitoring form should continue until 10 observation intervals have been completed.

To exemplify how the monitoring form is scored, a minute-by-minute description of what an observer sees during the first four minutes while observing the implementation of a consumer's (Patti) behavior support plan is presented in the following illustration (see earlier summary of Patti's plan as transcribed on the illustrated **Behavior Support Plan Summary Form**). For each of the four minutes, a summary of what occurs with Patti is presented, followed by a summary of how the monitoring form should be scored.

Example of How the Behavior Support Plan Implementation Monitoring Form Should Be Scored Based On Observations of Staff and Consumer Activity

Minute 1: Patti is playing with her video game in the living room with two other consumers present; there is no staff member in the living room.

Scoring: N is scored for environmental set-ups because even though she has a leisure material in arm's reach, there is no staff member present (remember, to score Y, all set-ups that should be present must be observed, and all set-ups that should not be present must be absent); NA is scored for antecedents because Patti was not observed to demonstrate repetitious talk; Y is scored for behavior to increase because Patti is engaging with leisure materials; N is scored for staff response to behavior to increase because no staff attention is given to her; N is scored for behavior to decrease because Patti was not observed to pull her peer's clothing; NA is scored for staff response to behavior to decrease because there was no behavior to decrease observed.

Minute 2: A staff member enters the room and praises Patti for playing with her video game.

Scoring: The scoring is the same as for minute 1 except that Y is scored for environmental set-ups because Patti has a leisure material within arm's reach and a staff member is present while Patti is in a room with her peers, and Y is scored for staff response to behavior to increase because a staff member praised Patti for engaging with leisure materials.

Minute 3: Patti moves to the corner of the room where there are no leisure materials present and begins to repeatedly say that she does not like Tomika (another consumer); the only staff member present spends the whole minute preparing snacks to put on a living room table.

Scoring: N is scored for environmental set-ups because Patti does not have a leisure material in arm's reach; N is scored for antecedents because Patti demonstrates repetitious talk (i.e., the antecedent behavior) but the staff member does not prompt her to engage with a leisure material when the antecedent occurs; N is scored for behavior to increase because Patti is not manipulating leisure materials; NA is scored for staff response to behavior to increase because there is no behavior to increase on Patti's part for staff to respond to; N is scored for the behavior to decrease because Patti was not observed to pull the clothing of one of her peers; NA is scored for staff response to behavior to decrease because there is no behavior to decrease (pulling on clothing) for staff to respond to.

Minute 4: Patti begins pulling on Tomika's blouse; the staff member physically interrupts Patti's behavior and asks her to go to the table and play with her video game; Patti begins to walk toward the table.

Scoring: N is scored for environmental set-ups because Patti does not have a leisure material in arm's reach; NA is scored for antecedents because there is no antecedent for staff to respond to; N is scored for behavior to increase because this behavior did not occur; NA is scored for staff response to behavior to increase because the behavior did not occur; Y is scored for behavior to decrease because Patti pulled on the clothing of one of her peers; Y is scored for staff response to behavior to decrease because the staff interrupted Patti's behavior of clothes pulling and directed her to another location (in which leisure materials were present) away from the other consumer.

Summarizing Results of Monitoring Staff Implementation of a Behavior Support Plan

The primary intent of systematically monitoring staff implementation of a behavior support plan in the manner just described is to determine staff proficiency in carrying out the plan. Because not every aspect of a support plan is expected to be carried out during every monitoring session (e.g., antecedents to behaviors to decrease may not occur, or the behavior to decrease itself may not occur during the period of observation), the focus should be on the opportunities staff had to implement the plan appropriately. More specifically, the percentage of opportunities staff had for carrying out aspects of the plan for which staff did indeed carry out the plan appropriately should be determined.

In order to summarize results of the monitoring session to determine the percentage of opportunities in which staff carried out the plan appropriately, the following summary should be conducted with the information recorded on the **Behavior Support Plan Implementation Monitoring Form**. First, the number of intervals marked as correct (**Y** on the form) should be summed for each of the categories of environmental set-ups, antecedents, staff responses to behaviors to increase, and staff responses to behaviors to decrease. Next, the number of intervals marked as incorrect (**N** on the form) for each of the just noted categories should be counted. The number of intervals scored as correct should then be divided by the sum of the number of correct and incorrect intervals, with the resulting quotient being multiplied by 100%. Note that any intervals marked as **NA** should be excluded from the count of total intervals before computing the percentage of correct implementation.

Once the summaries and calculations just described are completed, a determination can be made regarding the degree of accuracy or proficiency with which staff carried out each designated aspect of the support plan—that is, the environmental set-ups, antecedents and appropriate response to the antecedents, and responses to behaviors to increase and decrease. To obtain an overall figure regarding staff proficiency in carrying out the entire plan, all the correct aspects of carrying out the plan (again, **Y** on the form) should be summed, all the incorrect aspects (**N**) should be summed, the total number of correct aspects should be divided by the sum of the total correct and incorrect aspects, and the resulting quotient should be multiplied by 100%.

The following, completed **Behavior Support Plan Implementation Monitoring Form** illustrates how results of one monitoring session of staffs' implementation of Patti's support plan as described earlier are summarized. A review of the data summarization indicates that for this particular monitoring session, 60% of the intervals included correct environmental set-ups, 50% of the recorded intervals involved correct staff response to observed antecedents to the behavior to decrease, 29% correct staff response to the behavior to increase, and 100% correct response to the behavior to decrease. When considering all aspects of carrying out Patti's support plan, staff correctly implemented the procedures on 52% of the opportunities.

Evaluating Observed Proficiency of Program Implementation

A general guideline for evaluating the proficiency with which staff carry out a behavior support plan is what is considered the "*80% Rule*". That is, the goal to strive for is that staff will correctly carry out procedural components of a behavior support plan on at

Behavior Support Plan Implementation Monitoring Form

Consumer *Patti* Location *group home* Activity *leisure*

Staff present *Stan, Beth* Date *1/15/02* Time *5:30* Observer *Beckham*

Environmental Set-ups *during leisure times, Patti should have leisure materials in arms reach; she should not be in a room with her peers unless a staff person is present*

Antecedents
repeatedly saying the same thing; when she does this, she should be prompted to engage with materials (usually her video game)

Behaviors to increase
manipulating leisure materials

Staff response to behaviors to increase
give her attention (e.g., sit next to her) as much as possible; must praise or talk to her at least every 5 minutes

Behaviors to decrease
pulling on the clothing of her peers

Staff responses to behaviors to decrease
interrupt the pulling, escort her away from the peer and prompt her to engage with the leisure materials

Env. S-U	Antecedents	Beh. to Increase	Staff Response	Beh. to Decrease	Staff Response
1. Y ~~N~~ NA	Y N ~~NA~~	~~Y~~ N NA	Y ~~N~~ NA	Y ~~N~~ NA	Y N ~~NA~~
2. ~~Y~~ N NA	Y N ~~NA~~	~~Y~~ N NA	~~Y~~ N NA	Y ~~N~~ NA	Y N ~~NA~~
3. Y ~~N~~ NA	Y ~~N~~ NA	Y ~~N~~ NA	Y N ~~NA~~	Y ~~N~~ NA	Y N ~~NA~~
4. Y ~~N~~ NA	Y N ~~NA~~	Y ~~N~~ NA	Y N ~~NA~~	~~Y~~ N NA	~~Y~~ N NA
5. ~~Y~~ N NA	Y N ~~NA~~	~~Y~~ N NA	~~Y~~ N NA	~~Y~~ N NA	Y N ~~NA~~
6. ~~Y~~ N NA	Y N ~~NA~~	~~Y~~ N NA	Y ~~N~~ NA	~~Y~~ N NA	~~Y~~ N NA
7. Y ~~N~~ NA	Y N ~~NA~~	~~Y~~ N NA	Y ~~N~~ NA	Y ~~N~~ NA	Y N ~~NA~~
8. ~~Y~~ N NA	Y N ~~NA~~	~~Y~~ N NA	Y ~~N~~ NA	Y ~~N~~ NA	Y N ~~NA~~
9. ~~Y~~ N NA	Y N ~~NA~~	~~Y~~ N NA	Y ~~N~~ NA	Y ~~N~~ NA	Y N ~~NA~~
10. ~~Y~~ N NA	~~Y~~ N NA	Y ~~N~~ NA	Y N ~~NA~~	Y ~~N~~ NA	Y N ~~NA~~
#Y / #Y+N = *6/10*	#Y / #Y+N = *1/2*		#Y / #Y+N = *2/7*		#Y / #Y+N = *2/2*
%Y *60*	%Y *50*		%Y *29*		%Y *100*

Total #Y / #Y+N = *11/21* Overall % Y *52*

Figure 9-4: Sample completed *Behavior Support Plan Implementation Monitoring Form*.

least 80% of observed opportunities. Experience has indicated that if an appropriately designed behavior support plan is implemented with at least an 80% level of proficiency, the plan will serve its intended purpose of preventing or reducing a consumer's challenging behavior.

The "*80% Rule*" pertains to the overall level of proficiency in implementing a support plan based on the total number of correctly implemented aspects of the plan as described earlier. It can also be helpful from an evaluative perspective to review the level of proficiency of carrying out each of the main components of the plan (i.e., environmental set-ups, responses to antecedents, and responses to behaviors to increase and decrease). Often, certain staff will carry out some aspects of a support plan adequately, but experience problems in carrying out other aspects. For example, in the illustration with implementation of Patti's plan, the staff correctly responded to the behavior to decrease (100% of opportunities were correctly responded to), but were inconsistent in ensuring that the environmental set-ups were in place (60% of opportunities), and that her antecedent behavior was responded to in the specified manner (50% of opportunities). The staff had particular difficulties in correctly responding to Patti's targeted behavior to increase (only 29% of opportunities were correctly responded to). By evaluating which components of a support plan staff are implementing correctly versus incorrectly, a supervisor or clinician can determine the most effective supportive or corrective action to pursue with staff (see **Chapters 10** and **11** for an in-depth discussion).

Although the "*80% Rule*" is useful for evaluative and quality control purposes, it should be emphasized that an 80% level of proficiency is only a guideline. Authors of behavior support plans should determine necessary levels of proficiency on a case-by-case basis. In particular, for some types of challenging behavior and corresponding support plans, 100% proficiency may be necessary with some aspects of program implementation. For example, for some individuals who engage in dangerous pica behavior, and their support plan calls for staff to physically block attempts to ingest inedible items, the blocking must occur appropriately for every attempt. In such cases, any failure to block an attempt to ingest an inedible item could result in serious harm to an individual.

Although authors of behavior support plans should determine appropriate levels of implementation proficiency on a case-by-case basis, a general guideline is that procedural components of the plans should be carried out correctly on at least 80% of all opportunities

Additional Considerations When Monitoring Staff Proficiency in Carrying Out Behavior Support Plans

Using the **Behavior Support Plan Implementation Monitoring Form** in the manner described in this chapter represents just one of many ways to systematically observe and evaluate staff proficiency in carrying out support plans for challenging behavior. Many agencies as well as individual clinicians have developed other means of monitoring staff performance associated with implementation of behavior support plans. The point of concern here is that as part of an outcome management approach to working with staff to ensure effective prevention and treatment of problem behavior among people with disabilities, there must be some regular means of systematically and consistently monitoring staff performance.

When using the **Behavior Support Plan Implementation Monitoring Form** or a similar means of monitoring program implementation proficiency, there are several special considerations that warrant the attention of supervisors and clinicians. One consideration is when to attempt to monitor staff implementation performance. One of the difficulties frequently encountered when attempting to observe staff performance in this area is that it is often difficult to know when staff will need to carry out a specific program; challenging behavior among many people with severe disabilities occurs on an unpredictable basis.

Because of the unpredictability of many problem behaviors, it can be difficult for supervisors and clinicians to be present for observation purposes when staff need to implement certain aspects of a given support plan. This is particularly the case when attempting to observe staff response to consumer behavior that is targeted to be decreased. Generally, the only option for supervisors and clinicians is to conduct monitoring sessions during those situations in which the problem behavior seems to be most likely to occur. Determining situations in which a consumer's problem behavior is most probable can be facilitated if thorough assessments have been conducted regarding the events that tend to occasion the problem behavior and the function that the behavior serves for the consumer (see previous discussion in **Chapter 6**).

In contrast to difficulties in observing staff response to consumer behavior to decrease as part of a support plan process, it is usually easy to observe other aspects of program implementation. Environmental set-ups, for example, often represent parts of behavior support plans that should be observable at essentially any time, or during clearly predictable situations, for most consumers who have problem behavior. Similarly, there are usually many opportunities for staff to respond to consumer behavior to increase, such that it is relatively easy for supervisors and clinicians to select times to observe staff performance regarding this aspect of program implementation.

Generally, supervisors and clinicians should strive to observe staff implementing behavior support plans at times when consumers are most likely to display the problem behavior of concern

In addition to determining situations in which to observe staffs' implementation of behavior support plans, decisions must be made regarding how often formal monitoring sessions should be conducted. Although the frequency of monitoring usually has to be determined in large part on a case-by-case basis, there are several guidelines that can be helpful for determining the frequency of monitoring. The first and most important guideline is that there *should always be some routine monitoring of staff proficiency in carrying out behavior support plans.* As stressed repeatedly in this and preceding chapters, routine monitoring of staff performance is a critical part of an outcome management approach to ensuring adequate work performance among human service staff. In most cases (see following guidelines for exceptions), formal monitoring of staff proficiency in carrying out behavior support plans should occur on at least a monthly basis for every support plan for which staff are responsible.

A second guideline for determining how often to formally monitor program implementation is that *the more serious the consumer behavior of concern, the more frequently the monitoring should occur.* Consumer problem behavior that puts the consumer or other people at serious risk of harm warrants more attention than consumer behavior that is problematic in other ways but poses no risk of physical harm (e.g., behavior that is socially bothersome to others or interferes with a consumer's work or other adaptive functioning). Hence, for staff responsibilities associated with behavior support plans that address self-injury, harmful aggression, or life-threatening pica behavior, for example, monitoring of the staffs' performance in carrying out those support plans should occur frequently such as at least weekly.

A third guideline for determining monitoring frequency is that *monitoring should occur frequently when new support plans are initially implemented by staff.* It is important to ensure that when a new support plan is developed, staff can carry out the plan appropriately. In order to make such assurances, staff performance in implementing the plan must be monitored repeatedly once the staff have been trained in the program procedures. Actually, frequent monitoring of staff implementation of new behavior support plans should occur naturally as part of the training process that is conducted with staff once the plan is developed (see **Chapter 7** for elaboration on effectively training staff to carry out behavior support plans).

The final guideline for how often staff performance should be monitored is that *the more difficulties staff experience in carrying out a support plan, the more often their performance should be monitored.* When it is apparent that staff are not implementing a respective support plan adequately, then their performance warrants frequent monitoring relative to if staff are carrying out the plan proficiently. Frequent monitoring is necessary when staff performance is less than adequate in order to determine how to help staff improve their performance. In some cases, increasing how often staff performance is monitored will in and of itself have the effect of improving how well staff carry out a behavior support plan.

FORMAL MONITORING OF STAFF PROFICIENCY IN CARRYING OUT BEHAVIOR SUPPORT PLANS SHOULD OCCUR FREQUENTLY WHEN:

1) **the consumer behavior of concern poses a risk of physical harm**
2) **plans are initially implemented by staff**
3) **staff experience difficulties in carrying out a plan appropriately**

A Final Note On Monitoring Staff Implementation of Behavior Support Plans

The importance of monitoring staff proficiency in implementing support plans for challenging behavior has been stressed repeatedly. It should also be reiterated that as part of an overall outcome management approach to ensuring proficient performance among staff, monitoring is best viewed as a means to an end. Although monitoring can serve several beneficial purposes as noted in this and preceding chapters, the primary purpose of monitoring is two-fold: (1) to obtain information in order to support staff in continuing to perform their program implementation duties satisfactorily and, (2) to obtain information in order to correct inadequate performance when improvement in carrying out support plans is warranted. The last two chapters in this manual on Supportive and Corrective Management, respectively, describe how the results of monitoring can be used to fulfill these two critical functions.

Section V

Increasing, Maintaining, and Improving Staff Proficiency in Carrying Out Behavior Support Plans

CHAPTER 10

Supportive Management: Increasing and Maintaining Staff Proficiency in Carrying Out Behavior Support Plans

Preceding chapters discussed three critical steps of outcome management that are necessary to ensure staff carry out support plans for challenging behavior in a proficient and effective manner. Step 1 involves clearly specifying what staff must do to implement respective plans. Step 2 entails training staff in the specified procedures using competency- and performance-based training strategies. Step 3 consists of routinely monitoring staff performance in carrying out the plans during their day-to-day work activities.

The three steps just noted are designed to set the occasion, or make it most likely, that staff will carry out their duties associated with support plan implementation in the way the duties should be carried out. If supervisors and clinicians follow these outcome management steps, in many cases direct service staff will implement behavior support plans in a proficient manner. However, in the majority of cases, although these steps are critical in the overall process, the steps will not in and of themselves result in consistent and appropriate program implementation. Rather, the steps must be applied in conjunction with what is considered the *responsive* steps of outcome management. The responsive steps, which are also frequently referred to as *consequence* steps, pertain to how supervisors and authors of support plans *respond* to staff performance related to program implementation.

How supervisors and clinicians respond to the adequacy with which staff implement support plans for challenging behavior can have a powerful impact on how well staff carry out the plans on a routine basis. Attending and responding to staff performance represents a potent means of motivating staff to: (1) maintain proficiency in carrying out behavior support plans and, (2) improve their program implementation when such improvement is warranted. Corresponding to these two effects on staff performance, there are two steps of outcome management concerning how supervisors and clinicians should respond to staffs' program implementation. The first is *supportive management*, which represents Step 5 in the overall outcome management approach. The second is *corrective management*, which represents Step 6.

Supportive management involves responding to staff performance associated with program implementation in a way that encourages staff to continue performing in their current manner. Corrective management involves responding to staff performance in order to change or improve the performance. Hence, when supervisors and clinicians should use supportive versus corrective management is based on how well or poorly staff are implementing program plans. When staff are carrying out program plans in an adequate manner, then supportive management strategies should be applied. If staff performance is not adequate, then corrective management should be used.

The purpose of this chapter is to describe supportive management strategies for helping staff maintain consistency in appropriately implementing programs for challenging behavior on a day-to-day basis. The intent is to describe what supervisors and clinicians can do to make sure that once staff are adequately implementing program plans, they maintain the motivation and skills to continue implementing the plans in an adequate manner. Subsequently, **Chapter 11** discusses corrective management strategies for improving staff performance when program plans are not carried out adequately. **Chapter 11** also discusses how supportive and corrective management procedures can be used simultaneously. Simultaneous use of supportive and corrective management is necessary when staff are implementing some aspects of program plans appropriately but warrant improvement with other aspects of their program implementation.

Prerequisites for Supportive Management

Using supportive management to maintain staff proficiency in performing day-to-day work duties represents a critical set of skills for supervisors and clinicians. When supervisors and clinicians routinely respond to staffs' proficient implementation of programs for challenging behavior in a supportive manner, staff will almost always continue to implement the programs appropriately and effectively. Direct service staff also are usually appreciative of supervisors and clinicians who take a supportive management approach.

Before describing how supervisors and clinicians can apply supportive management strategies with staff implementation of programs for consumer problem behavior, two prerequisites warrant mention. Unless these prerequisites are consistently adhered to by supervisors and clinicians, supportive management cannot be effectively practiced.

Prerequisite 1: Supportive Management Must Be Practiced in Conjunction With Other Steps of Outcome Management

Supportive management strategies are not likely to help staff maintain proficient work performance unless the strategies are used in conjunction with the other steps of outcome management. Before supervisors and clinicians can respond in a supportive manner to proficient program implementation, they must know, for example, precisely what constitutes adequate program follow through (**Chapter 6**). Relatedly, unless staff have been trained specifically in how to carry out the programs (**Chapter 7**), there will be little for supervisors and clinicians to support; staff cannot be expected to demonstrate proficient work performance if they do not have the knowledge and skills to perform their duties adequately. Finally, unless supervisors and clinicians routinely monitor staffs' program implementation (**Chapters 8** and **9**), they will not know if staff are performing in a way that warrants support. In short, defining staff work expectations for carrying out program plans, training staff in the necessary implementation skills, and routinely monitoring staff performance are not only needed to set the occasion for staff to adequately perform their implementation duties as noted previously, but also to allow supervisors and clinicians to use supportive management successfully.

Supportive management must be practiced in conjunction with the initial steps of outcome management: specifying staff duties for implementing program plans appropriately, training staff in the skills needed to implement the plans, and routinely monitoring staff proficiency in carrying out the plans

Prerequisite 2: Supportive Management Strategies Must Be Sincere

A basic intent of supportive management is for supervisors and clinicians to inform staff that they are fulfilling their program responsibilities adequately, and to help them feel good about their work performance. When staff know they have performed well and feel good about their accomplishments, they are usually highly motivated to continue implementing program plans in a proficient manner.

There are many ways to let staff know they are doing a good job, and that quality work performance is valued and appreciated. However, across all the various ways, there is a basic requirement that must be met: letting staff know they are doing a good job and that their work is valued and appreciated must be done *sincerely*. People can usually tell when someone is insincere in their interactions, and the same holds true for direct service staff when a supervisor or clinician responds to their work performance. When supervisors or clinicians attempt to support staff performance but are not sincere in their attempts, the end result is not very desirable for anybody in the work place.

In one sense, noting that expressions of commendation or appreciation must be sincere would seem unnecessary. Being sincere in interpersonal interactions is a widely held social value. Nonetheless, the importance of sincerity is emphasized in regard to supportive management procedures for two reasons. First, unless supervisors and clinicians respond sincerely when attempting to help staff maintain proficient work performance, the attempts will not be successful. Second, despite the acknowledged importance of sincerity, insincere expressions of commendation and appreciation regarding staff work performance occur in many human service agencies.

There a number of reasons why supervisors and clinicians attempt to carry out supportive management strategies even when they are not sincere in their actions. One common situation is when supervisors or clinicians are instructed by their superiors to be supportive of staff performance, but they are opposed to or otherwise disagree with the instructions. To illustrate, agency superiors may mandate that supervisors provide positive feedback to staff on a weekly or other regular basis in an attempt to provide a motivating and productive work setting. However, the supervisors do not believe positive feedback should be provided to staff because, for example, they consider staff performance to be undeserving of commendation. In other cases supervisors believe that staff should not have to be provided with positive feedback to perform their jobs. Nevertheless, the supervisors provide positive feedback to avoid the wrath of their superiors. The end result is that the feedback is not provided very sincerely.

An in-depth discussion of problems with insincere expressions of commendation and appreciation, and why sincerity is lacking in various work environments, is beyond the focus of this manual. The issue is raised only to stress that if a supervisor or clinician is to use supportive management to help ensure programs for challenging behavior are adequately implemented with individuals who have severe disabilities, the actions must be sincere. If supportive management strategies cannot be practiced in a sincere manner, they should not be practiced at all.

Positive Feedback: The Cornerstone of Supportive Management

The core component of supportive management is providing feedback to staff regarding their performance in implementing programs for consumer problem behavior. In its purest form, feedback refers to information presented to a staff person about the adequacy of the individual's work performance. *Positive* feedback involves presentation of information that expresses explicit approval of the performance. Positive feedback is the most readily available, cost efficient, and arguably most powerful means of supporting staff in performing their work duties proficiently.

There are numerous ways in which positive feedback can be provided regarding staff implementation of behavior support plans. For organizational and descriptive purposes, the various ways are usually considered to represent either *verbal* (i.e., spoken) or *written* feedback. Both verbal and written feedback formats have relative advantages and disadvantages. The advantages and disadvantages, which will be summarized in subsequent paragraphs, should be considered when determining which type of feedback to use in a given situation with staff. However, there is an overriding guideline for deciding which type of feedback to present to staff that supersedes all the advantages and disadvantages. Specifically, *a supervisor or clinician should use a feedback method that s/he is most comfortable using and that has the most supportive effect on staff performance.* Elaboration on selecting the most desirable means of providing feedback in accordance with this guideline is incorporated within the following discussions of each type of feedback.

Verbal Feedback

Providing positive verbal feedback involves telling a staff member about the appropriate or commendable aspects of the person's observed performance. After a supervisor or clinician observes a staff person carry out some aspect of a program plan (**Chapter 9**), the staff person should be explicitly told what was performed appropriately or in an otherwise commendable fashion. In terms of encouraging continued work performance of a proficient nature, it is usually most effective if feedback is presented immediately after work performance is observed. Hence, when supervisors and clinicians observe staff implementing behavior support plans, they should strive to comment on the positive aspects of staff implementation performance as soon as possible. When it is not feasible to provide feedback immediately, the feedback should be provided at the first opportunity.

Although in most cases immediate feedback is preferred relative to delaying the feedback presentation, delayed feedback can still be an effective supplement to immediate feedback within a supportive management process. Staff can be very appreciative of supervisors and clinicians who periodically go to a staff person's work area to express commendation about some aspect of the person's performance that was observed during a previous time period. When staff know that a supervisor or clinician exerted special effort just to visit them in order to express commendation or appreciation for their previous work, the importance of the targeted work performance can become heightened. Such a process can also enhance staff appreciation of the supervisor or clinician.

Advantages of Verbal Feedback

The most apparent advantage of positive verbal feedback is that it takes minimal time, preparation, and effort. As such, verbal feedback is usually very easy to provide, and rarely interferes with other work responsibilities of a supervisor or clinician. A less apparent but equally important advantage is that providing verbal feedback involves a face-to-face interaction between a supervisor or clinician and a staff person. Face-to-face interactions are advantageous because they provide opportunities to observe how a staff person responds to the feedback, such as the degree to which the individual appears appreciative of the feedback. Observing how a staff member responds to the feedback presentation helps the supervisor or clinician determine future supportive management strategies for the respective staff person. Direct interactions are also advantageous because they afford the staff person an immediate opportunity to ask questions or otherwise resolve any uncertainty that may exist with implementing a behavior support plan.

Disadvantages of Verbal Feedback

The most apparent disadvantage of providing positive verbal feedback as a supportive management strategy pertains to use by supervisors or clinicians who work with staff over a large geographic area. This situation occurs most commonly in community-based congregate settings for people who have severe disabilities. For example, a psychologist may be responsible for providing behavior support services for group homes and day treatment sites across an entire county, or several counties. In such cases, providing frequent verbal feedback can be logistically difficult because the psychologist must travel relatively considerable distances to visit all staff who are expected to implement behavior support plans.

Although the disadvantage of verbal feedback as just noted is a concern in many settings, the logistical problems associated with serving a large geographic area nevertheless should not be interpreted as a reason to refrain from providing positive verbal feedback. As discussed in **Chapter 2**, effective behavior support cannot be provided from afar. Authors of behavior support plans and supervisors have to assume active roles in supervising staff implementation of the plans. Active supervision by its nature means frequent face-to-face interactions with staff. Providing positive feedback should be a primary part of those interactions.

Another disadvantage of providing positive verbal feedback in a supportive management capacity pertains to the skills of the person presenting the feedback. Although expressing commendation or appreciation about some aspect of implementing a program plan seems conceptually straightforward, the process requires an important set of skills. One relevant skill involves critically observing a staff person's performance in carrying out a program plan and identifying what specific aspects were performed adequately or commendably. This process requires sensitive observation skills among supervisors and clinicians. A supervisor or clinician can enhance the ease and accuracy of identifying what a staff person is doing well from an implementation standpoint if a monitoring process such as that described in **Chapter 9** is used.

A second set of skills that is required to provide positive verbal feedback as a component of supportive management pertains to presenting the feedback in a way that appears sincere to staff. Earlier the importance of being sincere when providing feedback was stressed. It is also important to *appear* sincere when commending staff work performance. Providing feedback in a way that appears sincere to staff requires creativity and interpersonal skills that cannot be assumed to exist naturally among all supervisors and clinicians, even if the individuals are truly sincere in their intent.

Difficulties in providing positive verbal feedback in a way that appears sincere to staff occur for a number of reasons. In some cases, a supervisor or clinician simply feels anxious or otherwise uncomfortable in certain social situations, such as interacting with a staff person in order to provide feedback about the latter's performance. Attempting to provide positive feedback when feeling uncomfortable often results in the feedback coming across insincerely or awkwardly. For persons who experience difficulties in interacting with staff in this type of situation, the best remedy is simply to work through the awkwardness and provide the feedback. In most cases, supervisors and clinicians will become more proficient in providing feedback with practice.

To help supervisors and clinicians become proficient in providing positive feedback effectively, it can be beneficial if they follow a general protocol for presenting the feedback. Because positive verbal feedback is often presented in conjunction with corrective feedback about a staff person's performance, a generic feedback protocol that can be used by supervisors and clinicians to respond to staff implementation of behavior support plans will be presented in the next chapter on corrective management.

Positive verbal feedback provided to staff must be expressed sincerely by supervisors and clinicians, and must *appear* sincere to staff recipients of the feedback

Another reason some supervisors and clinicians experience difficulty in providing positive verbal feedback has less to do with the supervisors and clinicians than it does with the staff to whom the feedback is provided. In some cases, staff are intimidating to supervisors or clinicians, and such intimidation interferes with the ability to provide positive feedback in a way that appears sincere. Feelings of intimidation occur, for example, when staff are older or more experienced than the supervisor or clinician, even if the staff do not intentionally try to be intimidating. In other situations, staff may resent the supervisor or clinician and deliberately try to intimidate or otherwise respond negatively to attempts to provide feedback. The latter situation may occur because staff have had bad experiences with former supervisors or clinicians. Alternatively, some staff simply resent a supervisor or clinician interfering with their ongoing work activities. The end result of each of these situations is that staff do not respond in a receptive manner to the supervisor or clinician, which makes the overall process unpleasant or awkward.

In most cases when staff do not respond receptively to attempts to provide them with positive feedback about their implementation of behavior support plans, the supervisor or clinician has little choice but to pursue the interactions. If indeed the positive feedback is sincere, and the supervisor or clinician persists in providing feedback, staff reaction usually improves. Most staff appreciate positive comments about their work performance and any negative reactions to supervisors or clinicians will diminish as the staff realize that the feedback is sincere. It is also helpful if supervisors and clinicians are responsive to staff reactions to their feedback presentations. Supervisors and clinicians should carefully observe how individual staff respond to different ways of expressing commendation or appreciation, and alter how they provide feedback based on what appears to be well or poorly received by staff.

Being responsive to staff reactions to verbal feedback is also helpful in overcoming a problem that arises when feedback about implementation of program plans is provided repeatedly to staff. If a supervisor or clinician says basically the same thing to staff across various feedback presentations, the feedback can lose its appearance of sincerity and consequently, its effectiveness. Supervisors and clinicians must be creative in expressing approval for staff work performance in different ways. Attending to how staff respond to each way can be helpful in developing new ways to express commendation as well as in revising ways that are not well received by staff.

A Final Note On Providing Verbal Feedback Effectively: A Clinician's Responsibility

For reasons illustrated in preceding paragraphs, many psychologists and other clinicians who develop behavior support plans have had unpleasant encounters when attempting to provide positive feedback to staff in congregate settings. Such encounters, and especially when they have occurred repeatedly, have resulted in respective clinicians forming an unfavorable view of staff. Various clinicians tend to view staff as being unconcerned about performing their job duties in a proficient manner, or being generally unconcerned about the welfare of consumers with disabilities. The result is that clinicians lose their motivation for working with staff to obtain compliance in carrying out the clinicians' behavior support plans.

When confronted with the situation just noted, it is important for clinicians to remember that direct service staff who are expected to carry out behavior support plans are actually part of the clinician's client or consumer caseload. As discussed in **Chapter 2**, direct service staff are as much a part of a clinician's caseload in a congregate setting as are consumers with severe disabilities and challenging behavior. Despite negative encounters with staff, whether due to lack of skills on the part of clinicians or to problems with the staff themselves, clinicians must persist in attempting to support staffs' program implementation. It is incumbent on clinicians to find ways to effectively support staff in carrying out programs for consumer problem behavior. Otherwise, there essentially will be no treatment of the problem behavior.

Clinicians must adopt the attitude that if staff are not responding to their attempts to support the staffs' program implementation duties, the clinicians are not fulfilling their own job requirements. Clinicians must alter how they are attempting to support staff, and persist in working with the staff. When clinicians accept the view that program plans are not working because staff are not implementing the plans appropriately, and believe that staff are at fault for the program failures, the clinicians have abandoned their professional obligations.

There are many ways clinicians can overcome problems with negative staff reactions to their attempts to support staff in carrying out programs for problem behavior. Most of these ways have been discussed in earlier chapters. For example, involving staff in the development of the programs, spending time in the staff work area, periodically helping staff implement the programs, and consistently involving staff supervisors in the program planning and implementation process can promote favorable staff responses to the clinicians. Although these activities can be effortful and frustrating at times for clinicians, they are nevertheless necessary. In short, it is the responsibility of clinicians to find effective ways to work with staff, such that staff appropriately implement program plans and consumers with severe disabilities and challenging behavior receive the treatment services they deserve.

It is the responsibility of clinicians to find ways to effectively support the program implementation duties of direct service staff; if staff are not carrying out program plans appropriately, then clinicians are not fulfilling their professional obligations

Written Feedback

The second general means of providing information concerning the quality of staff performance in implementing program plans for problem behavior is written feedback. In regard to presenting positive feedback as part of a supportive management strategy, this feedback approach involves commending or expressing appreciation about a specific aspect of staff performance in written form. There are many ways to provide written feedback, including brief informal notes, formal letters or memoranda, specially designed cards on which the feedback is written, and e-mail or other computer-based messages.

Advantages of Written Feedback

The primary advantage of written feedback is that it rarely entails the problems noted earlier associated with a supervisor or clinician being uncomfortable in providing positive verbal feedback. Often individuals who are uncomfortable telling staff about the good aspects of their performance have much less of a problem expressing the commendation in written form.

Written feedback is also relatively easy to provide, and especially when considering a supervisor or clinician who works with staff in different settings across a wide geographic area. Written feedback does not require the supervisor or clinician to actually visit each staff person in the latter's work site to provide the feedback. The feedback can be prepared by supervisors or clinicians in their offices and then sent to each respective staff person by mail or e-mail. Before written feedback can be prepared and sent though, the supervisor or clinician must observe staff carrying out a given program plan. Hence, visits to the staff work site are still necessary as part of the overall supportive management process.

Providing written positive feedback can be facilitated in many cases if supervisors or clinicians use a prepared form or card for providing the feedback. Many agencies as well as individual supervisors and clinicians prepare a standard form that is used solely for the purpose of providing positive feedback. Designated blanks on the form are filled in with specific information about commendable performance in carrying out a behavior support plan. The form is then sent to a given staff person through interagency mail. Forms that supervisors and clinicians have used in this manner include "*Performance Award Notices*" (that can be filled out and sent at any time), "*Performance of the Week*" (for sending positive feedback every week), and "*Exemplary Performance Notices*" (which are used for highlighting exceptionally noteworthy work performance). Numerous other examples of positive feedback forms exist (see **Selected Readings** section on **Providing Supportive Feedback**), with each type of form developed based on the guideline noted earlier in terms of what the supervisor or clinician feels comfortable with and what is expected to be well received by staff.

A final advantage of written feedback is that at times, staff are especially accepting of this type of feedback. In particular, when feedback is received in written form, it represents a permanent product for staff that reflects notice of their accomplishments in carrying out behavior support plans. Staff can keep the written feedback as a permanent reminder of the appreciation for their work. The importance of this type of feedback from staffs' perspective also can be enhanced if it is indicated on the feedback form that a copy is being sent to their permanent personnel file or upper management.

Disadvantages of Written Feedback

A major disadvantage of written positive feedback is that it lacks the face-to-face interaction component that is a part of verbally presented feedback. As such, written feedback lacks all the advantages of verbal feedback described earlier that are associated with face-to-face interactions between staff and supervisors or authors of behavior support plans.

Because of the disadvantage of written feedback due to lack of direct interactions, it is recommended that written positive feedback not be relied on exclusively within a supportive management process for enhancing and maintaining staff implementation of program plans. Written feedback should be a supplement to verbally presented feedback. One means of providing both types of feedback that can be especially effective in maintaining proficient staff performance is to follow up verbal presentations of feedback with a written summary of the feedback content. Similarly, periodically written feedback can be presented to staff at the same time that verbal feedback is presented.

Another means of supplementing verbal feedback with written feedback is to routinely present verbal feedback (e.g., daily or every other day) and provide written feedback less frequently such as on a monthly basis. The monthly written feedback can summarize or reiterate the commendable aspects that were observed with staff performance and previously described in a face-to-face interaction. This process can be especially effective for making sure staff are well aware of what aspects of their implementation duties they are performing well, and for impressing upon staff that such performance is highly valued and appreciated in the agency.

Written feedback provided to staff about their performance in carrying out behavior support plans should be provided as a supplement to feedback presented verbally in a face-to-face interaction

Formal Versus Informal Feedback

Both verbal and written feedback can be presented in formal and informal ways. In regard to verbal feedback, formal presentation usually involves a scheduled meeting between a supervisor or clinician and a staff person with the explicit purpose of commending the staff person's implementation of a behavior support plan. In contrast, informal verbal feedback is presented during the routine course of a staff person's work day, without requiring a special meeting.

The difference between formal and informal feedback presented in written fashion is essentially the format in which the feedback is written. Formal written feedback is typically presented on a specially prepared, performance evaluation form and is usually accompanied by a scheduled meeting in which the information is summarized for the staff person (i.e., the formal, written feedback is presented along with verbal feedback). Informal written feedback involves presenting information and commendation or appreciation about work performance in a brief note or on a short form that is not immediately associated with a scheduled personnel evaluation.

Both formal and informal methods of providing positive feedback, whether verbal or written, have relative advantages and disadvantages. Because the distinction between the two ways of providing feedback are most apparent when considering verbal feedback, the pros and cons of formal and informal feedback are discussed in subsequent paragraphs in regard to providing verbal feedback.

Verbal feedback presented informally is usually the most powerful way of helping staff maintain proficient performance associated with carrying out behavior support plans. Informal verbal feedback can be presented at essentially any time a supervisor or clinician observes a staff member performing some aspect of positive behavior support in an adequate or desirable fashion. As such, informal feedback can be built into the daily work activities of a supervisor or clinician. Supervisors and clinicians who are known for effectively working with staff, and in a way that staff find favorable, usually are quite skilled in providing verbal feedback to staff as part of their regular work routine. Consistent provision of positive verbal feedback on an informal or impromptu basis should be a goal for every supervisor and clinician to strive to attain.

A common characteristic of supervisors and clinicians who work well with staff and to whom staff respond to favorably is their frequent presentation of positive verbal feedback during the daily job routine

Although positive feedback presented in an informal manner is usually the most effective means of supportive management (again, in conjunction with the other component steps of outcome management), formal feedback presentations can be helpful. When feedback is presented in a formally scheduled meeting, the feedback often evokes more attention on the part of the receiving staff person relative to informal feedback that is presented multiple times during the work week. Formally presented feedback also is sometimes perceived as more important by staff than more frequently presented, informal feedback.

Because formal feedback can be effective at times due to the reasons just noted, it is recommended that supervisors and authors of behavior support plans supplement their provision of informal feedback with formal feedback sessions at regular intervals (e.g., monthly). It is also recommended that staff be made aware of the time schedule for conducting formal feedback sessions; staff should know in advance when the formal feedback sessions will occur. Such awareness can heighten staff concern and motivation for performing their implementation duties associated with behavior support plans in a proficient manner.

In considering the use of informal and formal feedback, it should be remembered that the focus is on *positive* feedback. The intent is to provide staff who are proficiently implementing program plans for problem behavior with frequent support to help them continue performing their implementation duties satisfactorily, as well as to feel good about their work performance. The focus on positive feedback (i.e., in contrast to negative feedback that denotes disapproval of some aspect of staff performance) is particularly important from a motivational standpoint when considering the recommendation that staff be informed in advance of when formal feedback sessions will take place. If staff regularly receive positive feedback on an informal basis during their work routine from supervisors and clinicians, then the positive feedback they receive during the formal feedback sessions will not be surprising to them—they have already been made aware that they are doing a good job with behavior support plans. Many staff will look forward to the formally scheduled feedback sessions because the sessions represent a rewarding experience.

The situation just described in which staff are aware that they are doing an adequate job and look forward to monthly or other regularly scheduled feedback sessions is characteristic of a motivating work environment that supports staff working diligently and enjoying their work. However, the situation is not commonplace in every congregate setting for people with severe disabilities. In many settings when staff are made aware that there will be regularly scheduled feedback sessions with their supervisor or other authoritative person in the agency, staff have apprehension about the meetings. Apprehension occurs due to staff being concerned about receiving negative feedback or other types of disapproval during the sessions. Such concerns exist either because staff have not been receiving positive feedback during their daily work routine, or because their previous experiences with formally scheduled feedback sessions have been negative or otherwise unpleasant.

Situations in which staff tend to be apprehensive about upcoming feedback sessions are not reflective of supportive management, and certainly do not foster a motivating work environment for staff. The apprehension staff experience about feedback sessions detracts from their daily quality of work life. The formal feedback meetings themselves also impede work enjoyment. The process may result in staff working diligently for a while, because staff will work hard at times to avoid negative reactions from their supervisor. Invariably though, this management style detracts from staff motivation to work diligently and proficiently in the long run.

In short, when attempting to support staff in proficiently implementing programs for challenging behavior among consumers with severe disabilities, supervisors and clinicians should minimize use of a negative or punitive management approach. Reliance on frequently presented positive feedback for aspects of work performed well during the daily job routine, supplemented with regularly scheduled formal feedback sessions that also focus on the positive aspects of staff performance, will result in much more success in program plans being implemented adequately. When there are aspects of staff work performance associated with program implementation that warrant improvement, then corrective management strategies can be incorporated within the supportive management procedures as described in the next chapter.

Positive feedback presented in a formal manner should be a supplement to informal, positive feedback that is provided frequently during the regular job routine

Positive Feedback Presented Privately Versus Publicly

Positive verbal feedback as part of supportive management can be presented to staff either privately or publicly. Private feedback involves a supervisor or clinician presenting feedback to a staff person in a manner in which no one else hears or observes the feedback presentation. Public feedback entails presenting feedback to a staff person in proximity of other people such that the latter individuals are aware of what is said to the staff member (e.g., during a staff meeting or within a group of staff in staffs' work area). The staff member also is aware that other people know about what the supervisor or clinician is saying to the staff person.

In most cases, people prefer to receive feedback about their work performance in a private manner. Although publicly presented feedback is well received by some individuals in some cases, this means of presenting feedback can be seriously disliked. When staff receive commendation for their work performance in front of other staff, the process can represent an embarrassing situation for the staff. Additionally, although sometimes other staff may subsequently offer their own commendation to the staff member (which is usually a pleasant experience for the staff person), at other times the staff may belittle or otherwise chastise the staff person. Staff may criticize the individual, for example, about being shown favoritism by the supervisor. The latter situation is generally not a pleasant experience for the staff person.

For the most part, positive feedback about staff work performance should be provided in a private manner. Public feedback should be used with considerable caution. When public feedback is attempted as part of a supportive management strategy, the supervisor or clinician who is providing the feedback should carefully observe how the staff person reacts to the feedback as well as how other staff respond. If there is any indication of a negative reaction by either the staff person or the person's colleagues, public presentation of positive feedback should be discontinued.

When considering the disadvantage of publicly presented feedback as part of supportive management, one exception should be noted. The exception is *third party feedback*. Third party feedback entails a clinician informing the staff person's immediate supervisor about the commendable aspects of the staff person's work in carrying out program plans. Third party feedback also involves telling representatives of upper management about the staff person's work accomplishments. Informing agency superiors about a staff person's noteworthy work rarely has any negative impact on the respective staff person, and frequently represents a powerful means of supporting the individual's proficient performance.

When agency superiors become aware that a given staff member, or group of staff persons, are doing a commendable job carrying out program plans for challenging behavior, the superiors represent another source of positive feedback for the staff. Often, the superiors will relay the favorable view of the staff work activities to the staff themselves. When staff receive positive feedback from upper management, the feedback can serve a potent supportive function for helping staff feel good about their work and to continue working in such a manner. The process also helps staff appreciate the supervisor or clinician who informed upper management about the staffs' work accomplishments.

Positive feedback concerning staff performance in carrying out behavior support plans usually should be presented in a private manner to staff; publicly presented feedback should be used cautiously

Supportive Management Responses Other Than Feedback

Although feedback is the most readily available and consistently effective means of supporting staff in working proficiently and feeling good about their work accomplishments, there are other ways supervisors and clinicians can respond to staff performance as part of a supportive management approach. These ways involve special *performance consequences*. When used in a supportive management capacity, performance consequences involve providing some type of special recognition, item, or activity for staff who have performed program implementation duties in a noteworthy manner.

The most common type of performance consequence is award programs. Many agencies have programs that involve awards for commendable performance such as employee of the month or year, outstanding teacher award, award for exemplary service, etc. Although these types of awards usually are not designed specifically for work performance associated with carrying out program plans for challenging behavior, the awards can be used to promote such performance by supervisors and clinicians.

Another type of performance consequence involves recognizing competent work behavior with desired items. The most apparent item used in this manner is special pay increases or related type of monetary award. However, because most supervisors of direct service staff and clinicians usually do not have access over agency personnel funds, money is not used very often in supportive management related to carrying out programs for consumer problem behavior. A wide variety of other items have been used in supportive management approaches though, including special gifts (flowers, clothing items with agency logos, etc.), free meals, and gift certificates.

A third type of performance consequence involves special activities or privileges. To illustrate, a number of agencies use trips to professional conferences and conventions as a means of recognizing noteworthy staff performance. Other agencies have provided special days off from work or specially designed flex schedules with which respective staff arrange their own schedule of days off for the month. Other common types of activity or privilege consequences include being relieved of selected work duties and having a specially reserved parking place.

Performance consequences such as awards, items, and activities or privileges have specific advantages and disadvantages when used in a supportive management capacity. The most notable advantage is that staff often are very appreciative of these types of responses to their work performance. Many agency personnel enjoy receiving special things or privileges as recognition for their work accomplishments. In a larger number of cases, staff are not as concerned with the special items or privileges as they are with the fact that a supervisor or clinician was willing to take the time and effort to arrange for staff to receive something special. Staff often feel their work is truly appreciated when a supervisor or clinician takes the time and effort to provide something tangible in recognition of their work.

The most notable disadvantage of special consequences is that they rarely work in isolation. To help staff feel good about their work and continue working proficiently, the special consequences have to be part of a more comprehensive approach to staff supervision. When special consequences are used as a singular strategy in an attempt to support proficient work performance, the consequences often have the appearance of being superficial or insincere.

Special consequences for work performance can help motivate staff to work hard and enjoy their work only if the consequences are used in conjunction with other essential steps of staff supervision

Another disadvantage of special performance consequences is that by their nature, they usually cannot be provided very frequently. The cost involved in providing special gifts or sending staff to conferences, for example, often prohibits their use except on an occasional basis. Relatedly, at a given point in time, special consequences can be provided to only a small number of staff even if many staff are performing their duties associated with implementing behavior support plans in a commendable manner. Only so many people can be employee of the month or year, or only so many people can be provided with reserved parking places. As such, these types of consequences can rarely be applied on a consistent, long-term basis with many staff to help support proficient work performance associated with carrying out programs for challenging behavior.

The Best Way to Apply Special Consequences as a Component of Supportive Management

In light of the relative advantages and disadvantages of using special consequences in supportive management, the following guidelines should be followed if a supervisor or clinician desires to use these types of consequences. First, as just emphasized, *special performance consequences must be used in conjunction with the other component steps of outcome management.* If special consequences are to be applied effectively to support staff in carrying out program plans proficiently, and to feel good about their accomplishments, the consequences must be applied after specific duties required of staff to implement program plans have been well specified and trained to staff, and staff performance has been routinely monitored in an objective and acceptable fashion.

If special consequences are not used in conjunction with the other steps of outcome management, not only will the consequences likely appear superficial and insincere as noted earlier, it is quite likely that the consequences will not be presented fairly. Without the other component steps of outcome management, there is no objective means to consistently determine which staff warrant special consequences for commendable performance. Often what happens is that the special recognition or items are provided to staff based on factors other than noteworthy performance, such as with whom a supervisor or clinician happens to be friends or otherwise has a particular relationship. When special consequences are provided based on factors other than clearly identified work accomplishments, then the actions are typically viewed by other agency staff as being biased or unfair. The end result is staff lose respect for the responsible supervisor or clinician, and their motivation to work hard or proficiently is clearly not enhanced.

The second guideline for applying special performance consequences as part of a supportive management approach is that *the consequences should be provided in addition to, and not in place of, positive feedback.* Because special consequences rarely can be presented to all or even many of the staff who are performing their program implementation duties proficiently, and rarely can be presented frequently, these types of items or events should be used in addition to feedback. As already stressed, the best way for a supervisor or clinician to support staff in working proficiently and enjoying their work is to routinely provide positive feedback. Positive feedback must be a regular occurrence in staffs' work place. In many cases, when supervisors and clinicians provide positive feedback repeatedly during the work week, and occasionally supplement the routine feedback with special consequences, a highly motivating work environment exists for staff. In contrast, if special consequences are provided when positive feedback is not routinely presented, there is little if any significant or long-term impact on staff work performance or motivation.

The final guideline when using special performance consequences is that *the consequences should be provided in a responsive manner.* Supervisors and authors of behavior support plans must closely observe staff reaction to presentation of special consequences, and base future use of these consequences on the observed staff responses. Attention should be directed to both how staff perform their program implementation duties when special consequences are provided, and what staff have to say about the special items or events. If there are indications that the consequences do not enhance staff work performance or staff do not like what is being presented (or the decision process regarding who receives the items or privileges), then the process should be altered or abandoned.

CHAPTER 11

Corrective Management: Improving Staff Performance in Carrying Out Behavior Support Plans

In preceding chapters, an outcome management approach has been described for promoting the proficiency with which direct service staff carry out programs for challenging behavior. If the procedures previously discussed are routinely practiced by supervisors and clinicians, treatment programs are almost always implemented in the manner they are designed to be implemented. In turn, individuals with severe disabilities and challenging behavior receive the supports and services that they are intended to receive.

Although research and application have repeatedly demonstrated the efficacy of the outcome management procedures described in previous chapters, the procedures are not fool proof. Despite competent and diligent efforts, supervisors and clinicians will likely face situations in which some staff do not carry out treatment plans adequately. Even though cases involving inadequate program implementation are usually the exception rather than the rule when the outcome management strategies discussed to this point are regularly practiced, the situations must still be addressed by supervisors and clinicians.

Addressing inadequate staff performance represents the final component step of outcome management. This step, or what is generally referred to as *corrective management*, is designed to be used when all the preceding steps of outcome management have been carefully applied yet certain staff fail to implement designated treatment programs, or implement the programs inadequately. Like the other component steps of outcome management, corrective management procedures have been developed through a considerable amount of research and application in congregate settings serving people with severe disabilities and challenging behavior.

Before describing how corrective management can be applied by supervisors and clinicians who develop behavior support plans, discussion is warranted regarding why some staff do not implement treatment programs adequately. An understanding of the reasons for inadequate staff performance in this area is necessary before corrective management procedures can be effectively used to improve program implementation.

Two Primary Reasons Why Behavior Support Plans are Not Implemented Appropriately

Numerous explanations exist regarding why problems occur with staff performance in human service settings. In actuality though, problematic work performance such as inadequate implementation of behavior support plans is almost always due to one of two basic reasons: either staff do not know how to do the job that is expected, or they do not want to do the job. In short, with a few exceptions (see later section of this chapter), staff fail to carry out programs for challenging behavior because they lack the knowledge or the motivation to implement the programs proficiently. In the most serious cases, staff lack the knowledge *and* the motivation to perform their duties adequately.

In order to improve inadequate work performance associated with carrying out behavior support plans, corrective management strategies must address the reasons for the inadequacies. Hence, corrective management must overcome staffs' lack of skills that are necessary to implement respective support plans, or provide increased motivation for staff to want to carry out the plans appropriately.

There are two primary reasons why support plans for challenging behavior are not carried out in the appropriate manner: (1) staff lack the skills to appropriately carry out the plans or, (2) staff lack the motivation to implement the plans appropriately

Corrective Management I: Overcoming Lack of Skills for Adequately Implementing Behavior Support Plans

When staff do not know how to appropriately carry out a given program for a consumer's challenging behavior, it must be assumed that the staff have not been adequately trained. How to effectively train staff to carry out support plans was described in **Chapter 7**. To review briefly, staff training should be *performance-* and *competency-based.* Performance- and competency-based training involves: (1) describing the program to be implemented to staff along with a rationale for the program, (2) giving staff a written summary of the procedures necessary to implement the program, (3) demonstrating how to conduct the program procedures constituting the program for staff, (4) having staff practice implementing the procedures in a role play or actual on-the-job situation, (5) providing feedback to staff regarding their proficiency in carrying out the procedures and, (6) repeating the preceding two steps until staff are observed conducting the procedures appropriately.

When performance- and competency-based training is conducted as just summarized (see **Chapter 7** for more detail), staff will have the necessary skills and knowledge to implement a designated support plan. When staff do not have the necessary skills, typically the training did not include all the steps just mentioned. Supervisors or clinicians become rushed at times due to competing responsibilities, or otherwise just do not take the time, to make sure each step of the training process is carried out sufficiently. In these cases, supervisors or clinicians must take the time to re-train staff who did not acquire the necessary program implementation skills, using the competency- and performance-based training procedures.

In other cases in which certain staff do not have the skills to carry out a consumer's support plan, the problem exists because the staff did not participate in the training. Various staff may have been absent from work when training was conducted, or assigned to other duties that prevented them from attending a training session, and the responsible supervisor or clinician was unable or forgot to arrange for the staff to be subsequently trained. This problem occurs frequently in residential settings in which there are numerous staff working with different work schedules, days off, etc. In such cases, arranging the time to make sure that all direct service staff are trained to competency can be a time consuming and labor intensive process for supervisors and clinicians. Nevertheless, the time must be directed to training all staff who interact with a consumer of concern if the staff are to be expected to adequately carry out the consumer's support plan.

In some cases, staff are effectively trained how to implement a consumer's support plan but over time the staff forget how to conduct respective components of the plan. This situation occurs most often when addressing a problem behavior that a consumer displays infrequently, such as only once or so a month. Because of the low frequency of the problem behavior, staff do not have many opportunities to practice implementing the consumer's program plan. The lack of practice can make it difficult for staff to remember all aspects of the consumer's support plan when the problem behavior does occur.

In cases in which staff have few opportunities to actually implement a plan such that it is likely they may forget certain parts of the plan, supervisors and clinicians should schedule periodic review sessions. The review sessions, which can occur as part of other regularly scheduled staff meetings or be scheduled explicitly for the purpose of reviewing a consumer's program plan, usually can be conducted with little time investment. The review typically needs to involve only a brief verbal description of the plan and perhaps a quick demonstration, along with the opportunity for staff to ask any questions they may have about implementing the plan.

When staff are expected to carry out support plans for consumer problem behavior that occurs infrequently, brief review sessions should be conducted periodically to help ensure staff remember how to implement the plans

Corrective Management II: Overcoming Lack of Motivation to Adequately Implement Behavior Support Plans

In preceding chapters it was emphasized that motivation involves staff working diligently and proficiently, as well as enjoying their work. When attempting to overcome inadequate performance in implementing behavior support plans due to insufficient motivation, corrective management must be conducted in consideration of both of these components of motivation. It is also critical that corrective management be implemented in conjunction with ongoing supportive management practices by supervisors and clinicians.

As discussed in **Chapter 10**, supportive management approaches are designed to enhance both the manner in which staff perform their work duties and the enjoyment staff experience during their daily work routine. Frequent presentation of positive feedback within a supportive management capacity promotes diligent and proficient work by staff. Positive feedback supplemented with other types of positive responses to staffs' implementation of support plans helps staff enjoy their work.

When staff lack the motivation to adequately carry out behavior support plans despite supervisors and clinicians routinely applying supportive management strategies, the lack of motivation usually pertains to the "working diligently and proficiently" component of motivation rather than the "work enjoyment" component. Even though the strategies are not sufficiently effective to promote diligent and proficient work by staff, the strategies are still often successful for creating an enjoyable, or at least a relatively enjoyable, work environment for staff. The latter aspect of motivation is still a critical prerequisite for successful use of corrective management procedures even when the work component of motivation has not been successfully addressed.

The significance of an enjoyable work environment for enhancing the effectiveness of corrective management relates to how corrective management procedures impact staff. As will be described in subsequent sections, by its nature corrective management entails at the least informing staff that some aspect of their performance is inadequate. In more serious cases, corrective management involves taking disciplinary action with staff. Both of these events—staff receiving information that their work performance is not acceptable and receiving disciplinary action—are not pleasant for staff. If these actions occur in a work environment that is already not very desirable from staffs' perspective (i.e., supportive management is not routinely practiced), the end result is a work environment that staff find most undesirable. When the work environment is especially unpleasant from staffs' point of view, there is little hope of staff working diligently to implement behavior support plans or of staff enjoying their work. There is also little hope of using corrective management to overcome staffs' lack of motivation to carry out behavior support plans appropriately in this type of work environment.

There are many reasons corrective management is rarely successful when applied within a work environment that is unpleasant or otherwise disliked by staff. These reasons will be noted in subsequent parts of this chapter. The primary concern here is that if corrective management strategies are applied when there are many other negative aspects with staffs' work situation, and particularly if supervisors or clinicians are viewed as responsible for the unpleasant conditions, the strategies are viewed as continuation of the existing negative aspects of the work place. As such, corrective management strategies draw little attention from staff and have little impact on how staff go about their work. Staff adapt to the negative aspects associated with corrective management in the same manner that they have learned to adapt to the usual unpleasantness in their work environment. In contrast, if corrective management strategies are applied within a work environment that is generally enjoyable and pleasant for staff, the strategies attract significant attention and usually result in serious attempts by staff to improve their work performance.

Corrective management must be practiced in conjunction with supportive management strategies that promote staff enjoyment in the work place

Steps for Using Corrective Management to Overcome Insufficient Staff Motivation for Carrying Out Behavior Support Plans

How to overcome problems with staff implementation of behavior support plans due to staff lacking the necessary skills to implement the plans was discussed earlier. In brief, performance- and competency-based training must be conducted (or re-conducted) with the staff in question, or brief review sessions must be provided. Such a process is straightforward and usually resolves the problematic performance rather quickly. In contrast, overcoming problematic performance due to staffs' lack of motivation to carry out support plans is usually a more involved process, and typically a more difficult undertaking for supervisors and clinicians

In one sense, corrective management strategies for overcoming insufficient staff motivation to implement behavior support plans can be conceptualized as a two-component process. However, actually implementing the two components in an effective manner can be a somewhat complex endeavor. The complexity occurs because the second component in the process depends on staff response to the first component. Additionally, the overall approach can become complex because sometimes the components have to be repeated with respective staff before improvement in their performance becomes apparent. Nevertheless, if the components are consistently implemented by supervisors and clinicians, the process is very effective for improving inadequate implementation of behavior support plans.

Component 1: Providing Diagnostic and Corrective Feedback

When supervisors or clinicians become aware that staff are not implementing a behavior support plan adequately, yet it is apparent that staff have the skills to carry out the plan (i.e., staff have been observed at times to implement the plan appropriately), the first step for improving the performance is to provide feedback to the staff. The feedback must be both *diagnostic* and *corrective*. Diagnostic feedback involves specifying for staff exactly what they are performing inadequately, or not performing at all. That is, the supervisor or clinician providing the feedback must first *diagnose* specifically what staff are not doing correctly in terms of implementing the support plan. Corrective feedback involves explicitly telling staff what they must do differently in order to correct the inadequate performance.

As noted earlier, corrective management inherently involves actions that staff tend to find unpleasant. Providing diagnostic and corrective feedback represents one component of corrective management that staff often dislike. Staff generally do not like to receive information that something they are doing, or not doing, is inadequate from a work performance perspective. Because of the negative impact such feedback often has on staff, and the fact that the feedback is critical to improving work performance, it is incumbent upon supervisors and clinicians to present the feedback in a way that removes or at least minimizes the undesirable aspects for staff.

Providing diagnostic and corrective feedback in a way that staff find acceptable coincides with a central premise of this manual. As stressed repeatedly, supervisors and clinicians should strive to provide a work environment that fosters staff working diligently and proficiently to implement behavior support plans, and to do so in a way that promotes an enjoyable work environment for staff. It is illogical to assume that staff can provide an enjoyable environment for consumers with severe disabilities—which is an integral part of positive behavior support—if the staff are working in an environment that is not enjoyable for them. Providing diagnostic and corrective feedback in a manner that staff find acceptable can have an important impact on enhancing staff work enjoyment.

Despite the negative features that are inherent in diagnostic and corrective feedback, research and application have demonstrated a means of providing such feedback that is well received by staff, or at least is not significantly disliked by staff. This manner of providing feedback as part of corrective management involves the following seven-step protocol.

Protocol for Providing Diagnostic and Corrective Feedback Regarding Staff Implementation of a Behavior Support Plan

Step 1: Begin feedback with an empathetic or positive statement

Step 2: Describe some aspect of carrying out the plan that the staff person performed correctly

Step 3: Identify each aspect of the plan that was not carried out correctly

Step 4: Specify how each aspect identified in Step 3 should be carried out

Step 5: Provide an opportunity for the staff person to ask questions

Step 6: Inform the staff person what will happen next in terms of observing implementation of the plan

Step 7: End the feedback session with a positive statement

Step 1: Begin the Feedback With a Positive Or Empathetic Statement.

When providing diagnostic and corrective feedback concerning a staff member's implementation of a behavior support plan, the feedback presentation should be initiated be saying something nice or positive about the staff member's performance. The positive statement may pertain to the staff member's overall performance (e.g., "You did a very nice job with many parts of this support plan"). Alternatively, the statement may be more empathetic in nature (e.g., "I know it can be difficult at times to carry out the plan with so many other duties").

The intent with **Step 1** of the feedback protocol is to begin the feedback session on an upbeat or positive note. A favorable or empathetic statement can help put the staff person at ease with the supervisor or clinician who is providing the feedback, thereby enhancing the staff person's ability to attend to the information that is provided. An initial positive statement can also reduce negative connotations that a staff member may have previously associated with a supervisor or clinician when the latter individual meets with the staff person to discuss the person's work performance.

Step 2: Identify Something the Staff Person Performed Well When Implementing the Plan.

To further initiate the feedback presentation on a positive or pleasant note for the staff member, the second step of the feedback protocol involves specifying something that the staff person performed well. Specifying acceptable performance not only helps to make the feedback pleasant for staff, but also serves an important supportive function (**Chapter 10**) in terms of encouraging the staff member to continue implementing the specified aspects of the plan in an adequate manner.

Step 3: Specify Aspects of Program Implementation That Were Performed Incorrectly.

Whereas **Steps 1** and **2** of the feedback protocol help make the feedback acceptable to the staff person, this step begins the diagnostic and corrective aspect of the feedback. Specifically, the staff person should be told exactly what components of the support plan were not implemented appropriately.

To help a staff person improve the way in which a behavior support plan is carried out, it is critical that the staff person know precisely what was done incorrectly. Often when feedback is presented to human service staff by people in authoritative or professional positions, the staff person is simply informed that the observed performance was inadequate or otherwise unacceptable. Such information does not always provide much help in supporting the staff person to improve the performance; the staff person may not be sufficiently aware of what aspect was incorrect. Specifying what was not performed appropriately helps ensure that the staff person becomes aware of what was not done adequately and what needs to be changed.

Step 4: Specify How to Correct Aspects of Program Implementation That Were Not Performed Appropriately.

Whereas **Step 3** informs a staff person what was not performed adequately, this step of the feedback protocol informs the individual exactly how to improve the performance. As with the preceding step, this step is often omitted from feedback provided to a staff person who needs to improve observed performance. Unless a staff person is explicitly informed how to improve implementation of a support plan, the individual may not be aware of precisely what needs to be done differently in the future. Without precise information about how to improve performance, a staff member may be aware that a program plan needs to be implemented differently and subsequently change how the program is carried out, but the change may not represent what should occur. A supervisor or clinician should make it very clear how the performance should be changed in terms of what the staff person needs to do differently.

In most cases, a verbal description of what the staff person needs to do differently will be sufficient to inform the individual how to improve the designated aspect of carrying out the behavior support plan. In some cases though, it may be necessary for the supervisor or clinician to actually demonstrate correct implementation of the procedures in question. Such a demonstration can usually occur in a role play situation.

Step 5: Provide an Opportunity for the Staff Person to Ask Questions Regarding the Feedback.

This step of the feedback protocol is intended to make sure the staff person fully understands which parts of the support plan were performed well, which were not performed well, and how to correct the performance. For some staff, when a supervisor or clinician meets with them to provide feedback concerning their performance, the situation evokes a certain degree of anxiety among the staff. Such anxiety can make it difficult for staff to listen and comprehend everything that is being explained about their performance. Hence, it is helpful if supervisors and clinicians specifically provide an opportunity for a staff member to seek clarity if necessary regarding the summary of the individual's performance adequacy. The best way to provide an opportunity to seek clarification usually is to simply ask the staff person if what was explained makes sense or if there are any questions.

Another benefit of providing a staff member with an opportunity to seek clarification about the feedback that was presented is that it can help demonstrate that the staff person's opinion is valued. Showing interest in a staff person's opinion, and sincerely responding to the concerns, can enhance a staff member's acceptance of both the feedback session and the person providing the feedback. Such acceptance helps make the entire process more pleasant for the staff person.

Step 6: Inform the Staff Person What Will Happen Next.

After providing the staff member with the diagnostic and corrective components of feedback, it is important to inform the individual about what will happen next in regard to observing program implementation. Usually this step of the feedback protocol involves informing the staff member when performance associated with carrying out a behavior support plan will be observed again in order to see how the implementation process is proceeding and to provide additional feedback.

The primary purpose of informing a staff member about when the next observation of carrying out a support plan will occur is to impress upon the staff member the importance of improving the designated performance. In many congregate settings, staff are accustomed to supervisors and representatives of upper management informing them about what is important concerning their job duties. Staff are also aware though that many supervisors tend to change their focus regarding what they emphasize with staff, depending in large part on whatever catches management's attention at a given point in time. Staff learn that if they simply go about their business as usual, the supervisor's attention will soon focus on something else, and the staff will not have to be concerned about changing what they are currently doing.

When staff are informed that their program implementation performance will be observed for evaluative purposes within a designated time period, the process helps to let staff know that the concern over this particular aspect of their work expectations is not transitory. In turn, knowing that their proficiency in carrying out a behavior support plan will continue to attract attention from a supervisor or clinician, staffs' motivation to improve their performance can be enhanced.

Step 7: End the Feedback Session With a Positive Statement.

The final step of the feedback protocol consists of providing an approving or encouraging statement concerning the observed performance. The intent is for the feedback session to end on a favorable note for the staff person. The statement may reiterate the positive aspects of the performance that were previously described, or simply express some type of approval for the staff member's efforts or willingness to listen to the feedback.

At first glance, the feedback protocol just summarized may seem to be a rather cumbersome way to provide information to staff in an attempt to correct problems in carrying out support plans for challenging behavior. In practice though, the process is really straightforward. Basically, presentation of diagnostic and corrective feedback in a manner staff usually find acceptable involves *letting a staff person know specifically what was performed well and not so well, how to correct the problems, ensuring staff understand the feedback, arranging for a time to observe future program implementation, and beginning and ending the feedback on a positive note.*

This means of providing feedback can be a powerful way to help staff improve their performance in carrying out behavior support plans. This type of corrective management strategy is also typically well received by staff relative to other common ways of attempting to improve staff work performance. Supervisors and clinicians should strive to become skilled and comfortable in using the feedback protocol. As with use of positive feedback as part of a supportive management approach, diagnostic and corrective feedback can be provided by supervisors and clinicians during formal feedback sessions with staff, as well as in an impromptu manner whenever a staff person is observed to be having problems in carrying out a given support plan.

Component 2a: If Performance Improves Following Feedback, Implement Supportive Management Strategies

As noted earlier, the second component of corrective management depends on staff response to the first component—that is, the staff person's response to the diagnostic and corrective feedback. In most cases, when staff who are displaying problems in carrying out behavior support plans receive feedback from supervisors or clinicians as described in the preceding paragraphs, staffs' performance will improve to adequate levels. When appropriate improvement occurs, the next corrective management component should be application of supportive management strategies.

As discussed in **Chapter 10**, the essence of supportive management is that supervisors and clinicians take active steps to support staff in continuing to carry out designated program procedures in a satisfactory manner. The most effective and readily available means of providing such support is the routine presentation of positive feedback to staff regarding their performance. Positive feedback that is sincere and that comes across sincerely lets staff know that their performance is satisfactory and helps them feel good about their work accomplishments. Consequently, when supervisors and clinicians observe improvements in staff performance after providing diagnostic and corrective feedback, they should provide positive feedback to the staff as soon as possible.

Once respective staff have improved their performance in carrying out behavior support plans and have received positive feedback for their improvements, then their work behavior can be addressed within a more comprehensive, supportive management process as described in **Chapter 10**. When the other component steps of outcome management have been routinely practiced by supervisors and clinicians, once staff improve their program implementation performance and such performance begins to be actively supported by supervisors and clinicians, such improvement will typically maintain.

Component 2b: If Performance Does Not Improve Following Feedback, Begin Disciplinary Action

In some cases, the performance of certain staff in carrying out behavior support plans will not improve even after diagnostic and corrective feedback has been provided (along with the appropriate application of the other steps of outcome management). When staff performance does not improve in such instances, the next component of corrective management is to begin disciplinary action with the staff person in question.

Every human service agency that provides congregate services for people with severe disabilities has a type of disciplinary action process. Although the specific procedures constituting a given agency's disciplinary action policy differ based on, for example, whether the agency is publicly or privately operated, or whether the agency is unionized or not, the essence of the various policies is the same. All disciplinary action procedures are based on a less-to-more punitive sanctioning process. That is, the first issuance of disciplinary action for a performance deficiency is less serious than subsequent actions provided for the same performance problem. The final and most serious disciplinary action is job termination. The exception to this type of graduated action process is when a staff person engages in an unacceptable activity on the job of a very serious nature such as abusing a consumer or stealing agency or consumer property. In the latter cases, disciplinary action often begins and ends with job termination.

Applying corrective management to resolve inadequacies in the way a staff person carries out a behavior support plan begins with providing diagnostic and corrective feedback and then: (1) if the performance improves, re-initiating supportive management practices or, (2) if the performance does not improve, beginning disciplinary action

---

Using disciplinary action as a means of responding to inadequate staff performance in carrying out a behavior support plan is considered the last resort within a corrective management approach. The purpose of disciplinary action is to negatively sanction inadequate work performance on a formal basis, and to inform the responsible staff that continued performance of such a nature will be followed by more serious punitive actions. Hence, from the perspective of both supervisors and clinicians who provide disciplinary action, and the staff person who is receiving the action, using disciplinary action in response to inadequate performance in implementing support plans is a serious undertaking.

Attempting to improve staff performance in carrying out a consumer's behavior support plan by using disciplinary action can be somewhat controversial. However, when examined objectively, the controversy is unwarranted because it is based on a serious misconception concerning the usefulness of disciplinary action in human service agencies.

A Pervasive Misconception About Disciplinary Action

There is a widespread view in human service agencies, both spoken and unspoken, that poor or minimally adequate work performance is to be expected among a certain percentage of an agency's work force. This view exists in human service agencies of all types, but is most prevalent in public or government-operated agencies. Although most agencies will take significant action to resolve the most serious performance issues, such as consumer abuse as indicated earlier, the agencies continuously tolerate other areas of poor job performance. Underlining the view that a certain level of inadequate job performance is essentially a given in human service agencies is the believe that disciplinary action cannot be applied to its ultimate end—that of firing a staff person—for anything except the most extreme cases of performance problems.

Many reasons are offered as to why human service agencies do not use disciplinary action, and tolerate repeated occurrences of poor staff performance. One reason frequently noted is that there are too many safeguards built into agency or government personnel polices that protect staff from being dismissed for continuously performing their jobs in a minimally adequate or even inadequate manner. Another common reason is that there are too many people in the administrative hierarchy of human service agencies who refrain from supporting a supervisor's attempts to fire a staff person. Lack of management support for a supervisor's use of disciplinary action occurs because management does not want to confront the disgruntlement or staff retaliatory action within an agency that often occurs when a staff person is dismissed.

For every explanation about why human service agencies tolerate repeatedly inadequate performance on the part of certain staff members, and refrain from using disciplinary action to improve the performance, there are strong counter arguments that refute the explanations. Most notably, there are sufficient numbers of human service agencies that do not tolerate inadequate staff performance, and quickly take effective disciplinary action to resolve the performance problems and when necessary, remove the respective staff from the agency.

Agencies that consistently provide services and supports for people with developmental disabilities that are of the highest quality are characterized by managers and supervisors who adopt an attitude that repeatedly inadequate job performance will not be tolerated. Such an attitude pertains particularly to those aspects of staff performance that directly impact consumer welfare, including implementation of consumer support plans. More importantly from the perspective of actually improving inadequate work performance, managers and supervisors in high quality agencies use disciplinary action efficiently and effectively.

Although disciplinary action should be considered a last resort for improving inadequate staff implementation of behavior support plans, such action is necessary at times and can be conducted in a highly effective manner

Guidelines for Using Disciplinary Action

As just indicated, disciplinary action can be a useful, albeit last resort, means of improving inadequate staff performance in carrying out support plans for challenging behavior. The degree to which disciplinary action is used in an effective manner depends on *how* it is used. There are four key guidelines for using disciplinary action effectively.

The first guideline for using disciplinary action to improve staff performance associated with implementing behavior support plans is that *disciplinary action should be used in conjunction with an overall, supportive management approach.* The importance of having a comprehensive supportive management process in place on the utility of disciplinary action was discussed earlier. Hence, the discussion will not be repeated here. The point is reiterated though because routinely practicing supportive management is a critical prerequisite for effectively applying disciplinary action. Disciplinary action must be a supplement, not an alternative, to supportive management as an approach to working with staff to ensure behavior support plans are implemented appropriately.

The second guideline for effectively using disciplinary action is that *disciplinary action practices must adhere to relevant personnel policies.* Essentially every human service agency has policies regarding the necessary steps for applying disciplinary action in response to problematic work performance. Supervisors must be familiar with their respective agency's policies concerning disciplinary action and closely adhere to the policies.

The importance of supervisors following agency policies when taking disciplinary action with a staff person is highlighted by a common scenario that has occurred in numerous human service agencies. Many supervisors have initiated various types of disciplinary action in response to staff performance inadequacies only to have the actions overturned by agency personnel officers or review boards. The actions are overturned (e.g., the actions have to be rescinded or documentation of the actions removed from a given employee's personnel file) because the supervisors did not follow correct procedures when taking disciplinary action. The actions are overturned regardless of the severity of the staff performance problems.

A primary reason supervisors have experienced difficulties with their disciplinary action undertakings being overturned is the cumbersome nature of many personnel policies that govern use of disciplinary action. There are often numerous steps for supervisors to follow, and a considerable amount of documentation mandated by disciplinary action policies. Failure to follow any of the procedural steps or acquire the necessary documentation can result in the disciplinary action procedures being overturned.

Many supervisors have viewed the numerous procedural regulations associated with disciplinary action as major obstacles to using the process as a means of improving inadequate work performance. Such a view is another reason the perception exists that it is extremely difficult to apply disciplinary action with many types of staff performance problems.

Procedural regulations governing use of disciplinary action exist in large part to protect the rights of employees from unfair practices by agency management. As such, the regulations serve a useful purpose. The personnel policies should not be considered as an obstacle to effective supervisory use of disciplinary action, but rather as a set of guidelines for supervisors to become familiar with and adhere to when considering use of disciplinary action. In many ways, following the component steps of outcome management helps ensure that supervisors adhere to relevant personnel policies related to disciplinary action (e.g., ensuring that work expectations are made clear to staff, adequately training staff in their work duties, objectively and consistently monitoring staff performance). Relatedly, supervisors can essentially task analyze the steps for instituting disciplinary action, and use the task analysis to guide their efforts.

Like most areas of work performance, supervisory use of disciplinary action in accordance with governing policies also becomes easier and less time consuming as supervisors become experienced with the process through repeated practice.

A third guideline for using disciplinary action to improve staff performance is to *obtain upper management support before initiating the action.* Earlier it was noted that one reason supervisors tend to avoid disciplinary action is that upper management is likely to overturn the action or otherwise not support it in order to avoid staff disgruntlement or counteraction (e.g, grievances) that often accompanies disciplinary action procedures. Such a tendency among supervisors is understandable. Anyone who has attempted to institute disciplinary action with a staff person due to repeated instances of inadequate performance only to have the action reversed by management has experienced the negative impact of this process. When a supervisor's actions are not upheld, the supervisor's future ability to impact the staff person's performance is seriously eroded.

To prevent the situation just illustrated, it is important for supervisors to obtain management support *before* initiating disciplinary action. Supervisors should inform management of the problematic performance, as well as their previous efforts to help the staff person improve (e.g., repeated monitoring and feedback sessions). It is also helpful if supervisors make it very clear to management how the staff person's poor performance is jeopardizing consumer welfare, as exemplified in failing to carry out a behavior support plan. It is likewise helpful if supervisors review the action that they plan to initiate with agency personnel representatives to ensure that they are adhering to the necessary policies. Reviewing the planned actions prior to implementation in this manner also helps to obtain the support of the personnel office for the supervisor's use of disciplinary action. In most cases when supervisors inform management and personnel representatives about forthcoming disciplinary action and obtain their explicit support, the action is less likely to be subsequently overturned even if a staff member seeks to have the action contested.

The final guideline regarding effective use of disciplinary action is persistence: *supervisors should persist in their efforts to use disciplinary action even if obstacles are encountered.* At times, even when the previously noted guidelines are followed, supervisors will encounter serious obstacles that impede or prohibit their follow through with disciplinary action. Sometimes supervisors make mistakes and do not follow all personnel rules closely enough, or upper level managers do not support a supervisor's use of disciplinary action despite earlier indications that they will support the supervisors. In such cases, supervisors should persist in their actions. For instance, if one attempt at disciplinary action with a respective staff person for failing to adequately implement a behavior support plan cannot be fully implemented, the supervisor should initiate the process a second time if the staff person does not improve such performance.

Persistence in using disciplinary action is critical from several vantage points. First, if supervisors follow the appropriate guidelines, their efforts will succeed more than they fail. Relatedly, after the first successful use of disciplinary action in terms of the action being upheld by management and personnel representatives, it is usually easier for supervisors to obtain support for future actions. Second, and more importantly from a performance improvement perspective, when staff become aware that a supervisor will persist with disciplinary action as long as work performance does not improve, staff become much more responsive to the supervisor's efforts. As staff respond to the supervisor's efforts to improve their performance in carrying out behavior support plans, then the supervisor can begin addressing staffs' implementation of the plans with a more positive, supportive management approach.

When considering the importance of persistence in using disciplinary action, it should be remembered that disciplinary action is a last resort for resolving staff performance problems within an overall outcome management paradigm. Disciplinary action is not a pleasant process for anyone in a human service agency and should only be used when all other components of outcome management, and particularly supportive management strategies, have been repeatedly practiced by supervisors and clinicians. Fortunately, if outcome management is consistently practiced within an agency, disciplinary action will not be needed very often. When it is needed though, it should be used appropriately and effectively.

The effectiveness of disciplinary action for improving inadequate implementation of behavior support plans is usually enhanced if: (1) the action is used in conjunction with an overall, supportive management approach, (2) the process adheres closely to all relevant personnel policies, (3) upper management support is obtained *before* initiating the action and, (4) supervisors persist in their efforts despite obstacles that may be encountered

Additional Considerations for Overcoming Inadequate Implementation of Behavior Support Plans

By consistently practicing the components of corrective management, supervisors and clinicians will have a systematic means of improving staff performance problems in carrying out behavior support plans. Consistent application of corrective management strategies represents a powerful means of overcoming both staffs' lack of skills and motivation for appropriately implementing the plans. In a small number of cases however, there are other reasons why staff do not perform their program implementation duties satisfactorily. In those cases, supervisors and clinicians must take different steps to improve staff performance.

Lack of Sufficient Numbers of Direct Service Staff

A basic prerequisite for the successful implementation of support plans for consumer problem behavior is that there has to be a sufficient number of staff to be able to carry out the programs appropriately. In congregate settings, lack of sufficient staff to adequately implement program plans is a commonly voiced concern. In a number of these cases, there really is an adequate number of staff, and the expressed concern is more of an excuse to avoid the effort involved in implementing respective support plans. In other cases though, lack of sufficient staff is a real issue.

When lack of sufficient numbers of staff appears to be a valid concern, supervisors and clinicians must address the issue if there is to be any reasonable chance of program plans being carried out sufficiently to overcome consumer problem behavior. In most such instances, clinicians have little authority to resolve the staffing problems. Staff supervisors usually have somewhat more capability of resolving problems associated with staff shortages. However, true resolution to problems due to insufficient numbers of staff usually must come from senior management within the agency.

When clinicians and supervisors are unable to resolve problems with insufficient numbers of staff, it is their responsibility to present the situation to agency executive personnel. Upper level managers should be presented with very specific information that illustrates the lack of sufficient staff to allow for adequate implementation of behavior support plans for agency consumers. The more specific the information in terms of illustrating the improbability or impossibility of staff being able to carry out specific plans at certain times or in certain locations, the more likely it is that senior managers will understand the situation. Such information will hopefully persuade management to make whatever short- and long-term changes can be made to resolve the problems. If management cannot or will not make the necessary changes, then it has to be openly acknowledged that prevention and treatment of challenging behavior among respective consumers is not likely to be successful.

The situation just described is not a desirable one for clinicians charged with the responsibility of developing ways of overcoming challenging behavior. This type of situation was illustrated in **Chapter 6.** Specifically, a dilemma faced in some agencies was noted in terms of a clinician developing the very best support plan possible even though the plan is too resource-intensive to be realistically carried out, versus developing a more realistic plan from an implementation perspective that is less likely to be effective. As also discussed in **Chapter 6**, there is no ideal solution to this dilemma. A clinician's only recourse is to make sure that everything possible is done to make agency management aware of the problem and its compromising impact on consumer welfare.

When it is clearly apparent that there are not enough staff to realistically carry out behavior support plans in an adequate manner, it is a clinician's professional responsibility to make sure management is well informed about the situation and the corresponding impact on consumer welfare

Competing Directions Provided to Staff

In some congregate settings, an obstacle that interferes with staff ability to adequately carry out behavior support plans pertains not to what staff are doing or not doing per se, but to the directions they are given. Direct service staff often have many people giving them directives or instructions regarding their daily job duties. Besides their immediate supervisor, staff may receive directions from their supervisor's supervisor, acting or covering supervisors when their regular supervisor is absent, and numerous professional or clinical personnel such as nurses, agency administrators, physicians, and social workers. Directives can also come from family members of consumers and advocates. At times these various individuals direct staff to fulfill certain duties that are in conflict to spending time with consumers in order to carry out the consumers' behavior support plans.

Duties that compete with staffs' ability to adequately implement support plans are multiple and varied. Sometimes staff are given explicit directives for example, to place a priority on updating certain types of record documentation, to stay with a respective consumer in the hospital, or to run errands to acquire supplies. Each of these types of activities, though important, can prohibit the capability of following through with the behavior support plans of respective consumers.

It is critical that direct service staff not be placed in the position of having to decide which directive or instruction is most important to respond to during their daily work routine. To avoid this situation, a collaborative team approach must be used in developing and overseeing the implementation of behavior support plans. Clarifying exactly who is responsible for supervising staffs' implementation of behavior support plans as well as other necessary work duties is also critical. For additional information on means of avoiding competing responsibilities being placed on direct service staff, readers are referred to the earlier discussion in **Chapter 2** on specification of supervisory authority.

Special Considerations for Authors of Behavior Support Plans

The components of corrective management described in this chapter can be used by both supervisors and clinicians to improve staff performance associated with carrying out behavior support plans. One exception however is the component involving disciplinary action. Clinicians and other authors of behavior support plans usually do not have the administrative or supervisory authority to implement disciplinary action with direct service personnel. The responsibility for initiating disciplinary action as a corrective management component in response to inadequate program implementation by staff usually rests with staffs' immediate supervisor.

Although authors of behavior support plans typically cannot conduct disciplinary action themselves, they can provide important assistance to a supervisor who must initiate the action. The assistance can occur in several ways. Most importantly, the clinician should work with the supervisor through each stage of the process, including when determination is made that disciplinary action is needed (e.g., the clinician should provide documentation of efforts to support the staff person and the continued problematic performance displayed by the staff member). The clinician should also assist in monitoring the staff person's performance to evaluate if the performance improves following the action. Clinicians can also participate in the presentation of the disciplinary action to the staff person, although the supervisor should take the lead in this step.

When disciplinary action is necessary to improve staff work performance associated with carrying out behavior support plans, clinicians should participate in the process with staffs' supervisor

Earlier in **Chapter 2** it was stressed that authors of behavior support plans must be involved to at least some degree in the supervisory process related to staff implementation of behavior support plans. Providing disciplinary action as one component of corrective management illustrates one important reason why a clinician must work closely with the staff supervisor. If a clinician does not work closely with a staff supervisor and it becomes apparent that disciplinary action is the only means left to improve a certain staff member's follow through with a behavior support plan, it is usually difficult to obtain the supervisor's willingness to initiate disciplinary action.

As discussed previously in this chapter, there are many reasons why supervisory personnel tend to avoid taking disciplinary action with staff. One way to overcome such avoidance and promote a supervisor's willingness to take disciplinary action is to ensure that the supervisor is involved from the onset of the program planning and implementation process. In this manner, the supervisor will be well aware of everything that has been attempted to support the staff member's appropriate performance associated with the program plan, as well as the problems the staff member is displaying and the corresponding need for disciplinary action.

When considering a clinician's involvement in the disciplinary action process with staff, it should be noted that many clinicians prefer not to participate in the process. In particular, some clinicians are concerned that if they are viewed by staff as being responsible, or even partially responsible, for the initiation of disciplinary action, their working rapport with the staff will be jeopardized. Such a concern is realistic in many situations. However, it must be remembered that the disciplinary action component of corrective management is the last resort in terms of attempting to ensure respective staff carry out support plans for challenging behavior in an adequate manner. If a clinician believes other, less punitive procedures may still be effective in bringing about improvement in a staff person's performance then those procedures should be attempted. At some point though, if improvement does not occur despite diligent efforts by the clinician, there is no alternative to disciplinary action. At that point, a clinician must fulfill expected professional responsibilities and help initiate more stringent action to bring about improvement even if the action is viewed by the clinician as a risk to the existing rapport with the staff person. In this regard, rapport between a clinician and a direct service staff member is of little value to agency consumers if the staff person persists in failing to adequately implement consumer support plans.

A major factor affecting a clinician's reluctance to initiate disciplinary action, as well as the reluctance that supervisors experience, is the impact disciplinary action has on staff in an agency. Of course, the desired impact is improvement in staff performance associated with carrying out behavior support plans. However, there is another impact of disciplinary action. When disciplinary action is initiated with a staff person there is usually an immediate response from the staff person as well as the individual's colleagues that the supervisor and clinician are being overly harsh or unfair with the staff person. This type of reaction within an agency's staff population is particularly apparent when the ultimate disciplinary action is taken, that of firing a staff person.

It is a rather common phenomenon that when a staff member receives serious disciplinary action, the responsible supervisor and clinician are viewed in a negative light by many staff in the agency. Staff tend to side with their peers when the latter are negatively sanctioned by agency management. This reaction occurs even if the action was well justified due to repeatedly poor performance by the staff member with whom the action was taken.

The negative reaction toward a supervisor and clinician generated by disciplinary action makes the job of a supervisor and clinician difficult and unpleasant. However, the negative reaction is usually short-lived. Although staff tend to feel sorry for a peer who is negatively sanctioned, staff also tend to respect supervisors and clinicians who will make a stand and take action against individuals who repeatedly fail to perform important aspects of their job. Such respect develops because staff usually understand that supervisors and clinicians have a job to do, and part of that job is to make sure appropriate services are provided by staff for agency consumers. Additionally, staff are typically aware that when a given staff person repeatedly fails to perform aspects of the job adequately, the job of the remaining staff often becomes more difficult. The latter staff essentially have to cover for the staff person and fulfill that person's duties as well as their own work responsibilities.

Staffs' tendency to develop respect for a supervisor and clinician who are willing to take serious action to resolve repeatedly inadequate performance is not an instantaneous occurrence. Respect develops over time as staff become aware that such action is conducted fairly and objectively. Equally importantly, respect develops when staff are aware that reliance on disciplinary action is an uncommon event by a supervisor or clinician relative to the usual reliance on positive, supportive actions. The development of respect for a supervisor and clinician by staff in this manner is one more reason why corrective management must be preceded and accompanied by strong reliance on supportive management practices.

Selected Readings

General Summaries of Outcome Management

Daniels, A. C. (1994). *Bringing out the best in people: How to apply the astonishing power of positive reinforcement.* New York: McGraw-Hill.

Everson, J. M., & Reid, D. H. (1999). *Person-centered planning and outcome management: Maximizing organizational effectiveness in supporting quality lifestyles among people with disabilities.* Morganton, NC: Habilitative Management Consultants.

Fleming, R. K., & Reile, P. A. (1993). A descriptive analysis of client outcomes associated with staff interventions in developmental disabilities. *Behavioral Residential Treatment, 8,* 29-43.

Green, C. W., & Reid, D. H. (1991). Reinforcing staff performance in residential facilities: A survey of common managerial practices. *Mental Retardation, 29,* 195-200.

Harchik, A. E., Sherman, J. A., Sheldon, J. B., & Strouse, M. C. (1992). Ongoing consultation as a method of improving performance of staff members in a group home. *Journal of Applied Behavior Analysis, 25,* 599-610.

LaVigna, G. W., Willis, T. J., Shaull, J. G., Abedi, M., & Sweitzer, M. (1994). *The periodic service review: A total quality assurance system for human services and education.* Baltimore: Paul H. Brookes.

McClannahan, L. F., & Krantz, P. J. (1993). On systems analysis in autism intervention programs. *Journal of Applied Behavior Analysis, 26,* 589-596.

Parsons, M. B. (1998). A review of procedural acceptability in Organizational Behavior Management. *Journal of Organizational Behavior Management, 18* (2/3), 173-190.

Reid, D. H. (Ed.). (1998). *Organizational behavior management and developmental disabilities services: Accomplishments and future directions.* New York: Haworth Press.

Reid, D. H., & Parsons, M. B. (1995). *Motivating human service staff: Supervisory strategies for maximizing work effort and work enjoyment.* Morganton, NC: Habilitative Management Consultants.

Wolf, M. M., Kirigin, K. A., Fixsen, D. L., Blase, K. A., & Braukmann, C. J. (1995). The teaching-family model: A case study in data-based program development and refinement (and dragon wrestling). *Journal of Organizational Behavior Management, 15* (1/2), 11-68.

Promoting Meaningful Activity Involvement

Evans, I. M., & Scotti, J. R. (1989). Defining meaningful outcomes for persons with profound disabilities. In F. Brown & D. Lehr (Eds.), *Persons with profound disabilities: Issues and practices.* Baltimore: Paul H. Brookes.

Jones, E., Perry, L., Lowe, K., Felce, D., Toogood, S., Dunstan, F., Allen, D., & Pagler, J. (1999). Opportunity and the promotion of activity among adults with severe intellectual disability living in community residences: The impact of training staff in active support. *Journal of Intellectual Disability Research, 43,* 164-178.

Parsons, M. B., Cash, V. B., & Reid, D. H. (1989). Improving residential treatment services: Implementation and norm-referenced evaluation of a comprehensive management system. *Journal of Applied Behavior Analysis, 22,* 143-156.

Parsons, M. B., & Reid, D. H. (1993). Evaluating and improving residential treatment during group leisure situations: A program replication and refinement. *Research in Developmental Disabilities, 14,* 67-85.

Reid, D. H., & Parsons, M. B. (1990). *Providing active treatment in residential environments for persons with severe handicaps: A working manual for practitioners, supervisors and evaluators.* Morganton, NC: Habilitative Management Consultants

Reid, D. H., Parsons, M. B., & Green, C. W. (2001). Evaluating the functional utility of congregate day treatment activities for adults with severe disabilities. *American Journal on Mental Retardation, 106,* 460-469.

Sturmey, P. (1995). Evaluating and improving residential treatment during group leisure situations: An independent replication. *Behavioral Interventions, 10,* 59-67.

Determining Consumer Activity Preferences

Belfiore, P. J., & Toro-Zambrana, W. (1994). *Recognizing choices in community settings by people with significant disabilities.* Washington, D.C.: American Association on Mental Retardation.

Green, C. W., Reid, D. H., Canipe, V. S., & Gardner, S. M. (1991). A comprehensive evaluation of reinforcer identification processes for persons with profound multiple handicaps. *Journal of Applied Behavior Analysis, 24,* 537-552.

Hughes, C., Pitkin, S. E., & Lorden, S. W. (1998). Assessing preferences and choices of persons with severe and profound mental retardation. *Education and Training in Mental Retardation and Developmental Disabilities, 33,* 299-316.

Lancioni, G. E., O'Reilly, M. G., & Emerson, E. (1996). A review of choice research with people with severe and profound developmental disabilities. *Research in Developmental Disabilities. 17,* 391-411.

Lohrmann-O'Rourke, S., & Browder, D. M. (1998). Empirically based methods to assess the preferences of individuals with severe disabilities. *American Journal on Mental Retardation, 103,* 146-161.

Newton, J. S., Ard, W. R., & Homer, R. H. (1993). Validating predicted activity preferences of individuals with severe disabilities. *Journal of Applied Behavior Analysis, 26,* 239-245.

Parsons, M. B., Harper, V. N., Jensen, J. M., & Reid, D. H. (1997). Assisting older adults with severe disabilities in expressing leisure preferences: A protocol for determining choice-making skills. *Research in Developmental Disabilities, 18,* 113-126.

Reid, D. H., Everson, J. M., & Green, C. W. (1999). A systematic evaluation of preferences identified through person-centered planning for people with profound multiple disabilities. *Journal of Applied Behavior Analysis, 32,* 467-477.

Developing Quality Behavior Support Plans

Bambara, L. M., & Knoster, T. (1998). *Designing positive behavioral support plans.* Washington, D.C.: American Association on Mental Retardation.

Carr, E. G., Horner, R. H., Turnbull, A. P., Marquis, J. G., McLaughlin, D. M., McAtee, M. L., Smith, C. E., Ryan, K. A., Ruef, M. B., & Doolabh, A. (1999). *Positive behavior support for people with developmental disabilities: A research synthesis.* Washington, D.C.: American Association on Mental Retardation.

Carr, E. G., Levin, L., McConnachie, G., Carlson, J. I., Kemp, D. C., & Smith, C. E. (1994). *Communication-based intervention for problem behavior: A user 's guide for producing positive change.* Baltimore: Paul H. Brookes.

Dunlap, G., Hieneman, M., Knoster, T., Fox. L., Anderson, J., & Albin, R. W. (2000). Essential elements of inservice training in positive behavior support. *Journal of Positive Behavior Interventions, 2,* 22-32.

Durand, V. M. (1990). *Severe behavior problems: A functional communication training approach.* New York: Guilford Press.

Koegel, L. R., Koegel, R. L., & Dunlap, G. (1996). *Positive behavioral support: Including people with difficult behavior in the community.* Baltimore: Paul H Brookes.

Luiselli, J. K., & Cameron, M. J. (Eds.). (1998). *Antecedent control: Innovative approaches to behavioral support.* Baltimore: Paul H. Brookes.

O'Neill, R. E., Horner, R. H., Albin, R. W., Storey, K., & Sprague, J. R. (1990). *Functional analysis of problem behavior: A practical assessment guide.* Sycamore, IL: Sycamore Press.

O'Neill, R. E., Horner, R. H., Albin, R. W., Storey, K., Sprague, J. R., & Newton, J. S. (1997). *Functional analysis of problem behavior: From effective assessment to effective support.* Belmont, CA: Wadsworth.

Reichle, J., & Wacker, D. (Eds.). (1993). *Communicative alternatives to challenging behavior: Integrating functional assessment and intervention strategies.* Baltimore: Paul H. Brookes.

Reid, D. H., Parsons, M. B., Rotholz, D. A., Braswell, B. A., & Morris, L. A. (in press). *The Carolina Curriculum on Positive Behavior Support: Supervisory Edition.* Washington, D. C.: American Association on Mental Retardation.

Repp, A. C., & Horner, R. H. (Eds.). (1999). *Functional analysis of problem behavior: From effective assessment to effective support.* Belmont, CA: Wadsworth.

Scotti, J. R., & Meyer, L. H. (Eds.). (1999). *Behavioral intervention: Principles, models, and practices.* Baltimore: Paul H. Brookes.

Providing Supportive Feedback

Allen, J., & Snyder, G. (1990). *1 saw what you did and I know who you are: Giving & receiving recognition.* Tucker, GA: Performance Management Publications.

Alavosius, M. P., & Sulzer-Azaroff, B. (1990). Acquisition and maintenance of health-care routines as a function of feedback density. *Journal of Applied Behavior Analysis, 23,* 151-162.

Horner, R. H., Thompsen, L. S., & Storey, K. (1990). Effects of case manager feedback on the quality of individual habilitation plan objectives. *Mental Retardation, 28,* 227-231.

McGimsey, J. F., Greene, B. F., & Lutzker, J. R. (1995). Competence in aspects of behavioral treatment and consultation: Implications for service delivery and graduate training. *Journal of Applied Behavior Analysis, 28,* 301-315.

Parsons, M. B., & Reid, D. H. (1995). Training residential supervisors to provide feedback for maintaining staff teaching skills with people who have severe disabilities. *Journal of Applied Behavior Analysis,* 28, 317-322.

Reid, D. H., & Parsons, M. B. (1995). *Motivating human service staff: Supervisory strategies for maximizing work effort and work enjoyment.* Morganton, NC: Habilitative Management Consultants.

Reid, D. H., Parsons, M. B., & Green, C. W. (1989). *Staff management in human services: Behavioral research and application.* Springfield, IL: Charles C. Thomas.

Appendix

Behavior Support Plan Implementation Monitoring Form For Monitoring and Evaluating Staff Proficiency in Carrying Out Behavior Support Plans

Behavior Support Plan Implementation Monitoring Form

Consumer ________ Location __________ Activity ____________________

Staff present ________________ Date ______ Time ______ Observer __________

Environmental Set-ups

Antecedents

Behaviors to increase

Staff response to behaviors to increase

Behaviors to decrease

Staff responses to behaviors to decrease

Env. S-U	Antecedents	Beh. to Increase	Staff Response	Beh. to Decrease	Staff Response
1. Y N NA	Y N NA	Y N NA	Y N NA	Y N NA	Y N NA
2. Y N NA	Y N NA	Y N NA	Y N NA	Y N NA	Y N NA
3. Y N NA	Y N NA	Y N NA	Y N NA	Y N NA	Y N NA
4. Y N NA	Y N NA	Y N NA	Y N NA	Y N NA	Y N NA
5. Y N NA	Y N NA	Y N NA	Y N NA	Y N NA	Y N NA
6. Y N NA	Y N NA	Y N NA	Y N NA	Y N NA	Y N NA
7. Y N NA	Y N NA	Y N NA	Y N NA	Y N NA	Y N NA
8. Y N NA	Y N NA	Y N NA	Y N NA	Y N NA	Y N NA
9. Y N NA	Y N NA	Y N NA	Y N NA	Y N NA	Y N NA
10. Y N NA	Y N NA	Y N NA	Y N NA	Y N NA	Y N NA
#Y / #Y + N = ____	#Y / #Y + N = ____		#Y / #Y + N = ____		#Y / #Y + N = ____
%Y ____	%Y ____		%Y ____		%Y ____

Total #Y / #Y + N = ______ Overall % Y ______

INDEX

TO ORDER ADDITIONAL COPIES OF

WORKING WITH STAFF TO OVERCOME CHALLENGING BEHAVIOR AMONG PEOPLE WHO HAVE SEVERE DISABILITIES

CONTACT

HABILITATIVE MANAGEMENT CONSULTANTS, INC.

P.O. BOX 2295
MORGANTON, NC 28680
PHONE: (828) 432-0030; FAX: (828) 433-8889

* * * * * * * * * * * * * * * * * * * *

HUMAN SERVICE AGENCIES, INSTRUCTORS

Discounts on this manual are available for bulk purchases. Write or call for information on discount purchases.